THE 12-MINUTE ATHLETE

THE 12-MINUTE ATHLETE

GET FITTER, FASTER, AND STRONGER USING HIIT AND YOUR BODYWEIGHT

KRISTA STRYKER

Tiller Press

New York   London   Toronto   Sydney   New Delhi

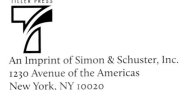

An Imprint of Simon & Schuster, Inc.
1230 Avenue of the Americas
New York, NY 10020

First Tiller Press trade paperback edition March 2020

TILLER PRESS and colophon are trademarks of Simon & Schuster, Inc.

For information about special discounts for bulk purchases, please contact Simon & Schuster Special Sales at 1-866-506-1949 or business@simonandschuster.com.

The Simon & Schuster Speakers Bureau can bring authors to your live event. For more information or to book an event, contact the Simon & Schuster Speakers Bureau at 1-866-248-3049 or visit our website at www.simonspeakers.com.

Photographs on pages xii, 40, 45, 46, 47, 48, 49, 50, 51, 55, 57, 58, 59, 60, 61, 64, 66, 67, 68, 69, 70, 71, 72, 75, 88, 95, 99, 100, 105, 110, 111, 112, 113, 115, 117, 118, 119, 120, 121, 123, 124, 127, 128, 138, 139, 140, 143, 147, 148, 149, 150, 151, 152, 153, 156, 159, and 242 by Tamara Muth-King.
Photographs on pages 52, 53, 54, 56, 65, 74, 76, 77, 79, 80, 81, 82, 85, 86, 87, 90, 91, 92, 103, 104, 106, 107, 114, 115, 116, 119, 125, 126, 127, 129, 130, 131, 132, 133, 134, 137, 138, 144, 145, 149, 151, 154, 155, 171, 172, 173, and 174 by Drew Doyon.
Photographs on pages 42 and 135 by Katana Triplett.

Interior design by Jennifer Chung

Manufactured in the United States of America

10 9 8 7 6 5 4 3 2 1

Library of Congress Cataloging-in-Publication Data
Names: Stryker, Krista, author.
Title: The 12-minute athlete : get fitter, faster, and stronger using HIIT and your bodyweight / Krista Stryker.
Other titles: Twelve-minute athlete : get fitter, faster, and stronger using high intensity interval training and your bodyweight
Description: First Tiller Press trade paperback edition. | New York : Tiller Press, 2020. | Includes index.
Identifiers: LCCN 2019049593 (print) | LCCN 2019049594 (ebook) | ISBN 9781982136482 (paperback) | ISBN 9781982136499 (ebook)
Subjects: LCSH: Interval training. | Weight training. | Nutrition.
Classification: LCC GV481 .S769 2020 (print) | LCC GV481 (ebook) | DDC 613.7—dc23
LC record available at https://lccn.loc.gov/2019049593
LC ebook record available at https://lccn.loc.gov/2019049594

ISBN 978-1-9821-3648-2
ISBN 978-1-9821-3649-9 (ebook)

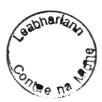

To my parents, for showing me the joy of an active lifestyle

CONTENTS

IT'S TIME TO DITCH YOUR EXCUSES— FOR GOOD

What if I told you that you could ditch your gym membership and give up using weights or cardio machines forever—and still get in the best shape of your life? And what if I also told you that you could get your *entire* workout done in under twenty minutes—and get fitter, faster, and stronger than you ever thought possible?

To most people that sounds crazy—maybe even impossible. Most people think they have to spend hours in a gym, five days a week, to reach their fitness goals. But most people are wrong.

Most health-conscious people are used to equating exercise with long and boring gym sessions that last at least an hour, if not more. And I am no stranger to this mind-set—I used to be a part of this "long workouts are better" camp, too, back in the days when I'd force myself to spend upward of two hours a day meticulously getting in my cardio and strength training workouts, only to feel like it was never enough. I absolutely hated it, but I did it anyway. I thought that spending more time exercising was the only way to get into great shape.

But just because you are used to something doesn't mean you should accept that's how it has to be.

Here's the truth: longer workouts aren't necessarily better. In fact, longer workouts can actually be *less* effective than shorter ones for many reasons. And your long workouts may be the real reason that you are not in the incredible shape you want to be in, or the reason that you can't seem to keep a consistent workout schedule.

That's where high-intensity interval training (HIIT) comes in.

Let's make things clear—HIIT is not a magic pill. It isn't exactly easy, either. In fact, it's actually really, really tough. During HIIT-style workouts, you are going to have to work harder than you ever imagined. In order to meet your goals, you're going to have to constantly push yourself past your comfort zone. It's not for the weak of heart. But if you can push yourself, if you can push past those mental blocks and tell yourself you can do this, HIIT can get you in better shape than ever before—and all in less than fifteen minutes. No gym required.

OLD SCHOOL STYLE

You don't need any equipment to get stronger and fitter—but if you want to add a few tools to your training regimen, you can use a basic pull-up bar, a set of parallel bars (or a dip bar equivalent), a plyo box or sturdy elevated surface (a bench or some stairs work perfectly), and a jump rope. Although these pieces of equipment are probably the least used at the gym (and seriously, what typical gym even has a jump rope?), they are by far the most versatile and most effective pieces of workout equipment you will ever use.

Simple metal bars offer a lifetime of challenges, from pull-ups, to triceps dips, to leg raises, to more advanced exercises like muscle-ups and the elusive one-arm pull-up. These types of exercises are typically known as calisthenics or bodyweight exercises. When doing them, you utilize your own bodyweight along with gravity to constantly challenge your fitness level. Calisthenics exercises have a lot in common with gymnastics exercises, but unlike formal gymnastics, anyone of any age, fitness level, or ability can benefit from adding calisthenics exercises to their regular workout routine.

When it comes to getting your heart rate up, the humble jump rope will do more to keep you coordinated and athletically fit than any machine at the gym will. It also functions as a portable piece of cardio equipment you can take with you anywhere and everywhere (unlike a treadmill or elliptical machine).

Using your own bodyweight, in addition to these simple pieces of equipment used by calisthenics masters, means you'll have enough to keep pushing the boundaries of your fitness for life.

NO MORE EXCUSES

I am about to tell you how you can get in the best shape of your life using nothing more than your own bodyweight, a couple of bars, and a five-dollar jump rope. Whether your personal fitness goal is to get stronger and leaner, to do your first pull-up, to look better naked, or to live a longer, healthier, and happier life and be able to keep up with your grandchildren, you now have the tools in front of you to reach every goal you've ever dreamed of.

If you follow my plan, you will achieve the impossible and become the athlete you were always meant to be. But I can't force you to work out—ultimately it is up to you to put in the hard work.

So my question for you is, *Are you ready to ditch your excuses for good and get in the best shape of your life?*

I hope so.

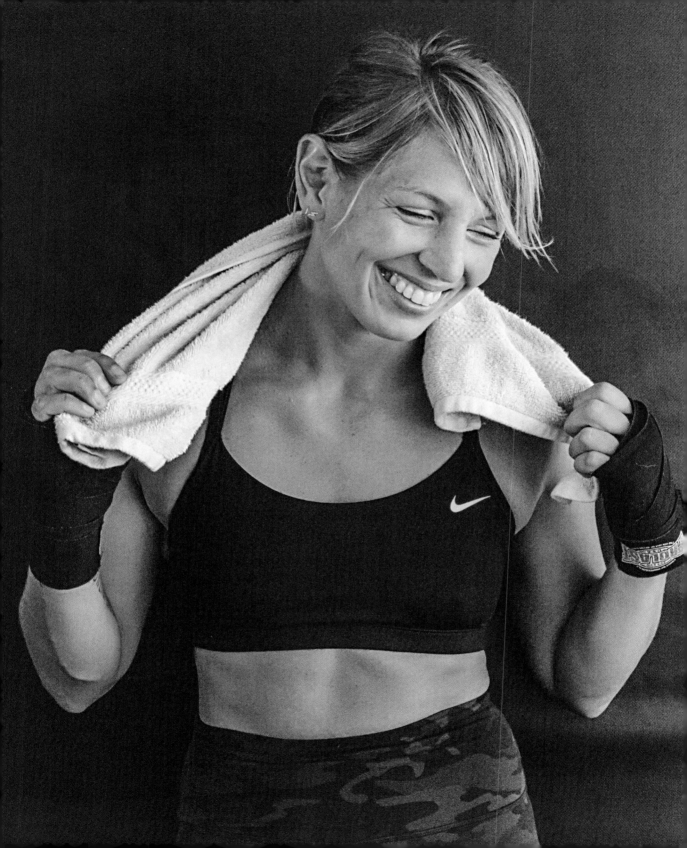

1.

GET IN THE BEST SHAPE OF YOUR LIFE

If you have a body, you are an athlete.
—BILL BOWERMAN

MY STORY: HOW I GOT HERE AND WHY ANYBODY CAN DO THESE WORKOUTS

Growing up, I thought the exercise gene had "skipped" me.

I come from a fairly active family—my dad, who, as of the writing of this book is about to celebrate his seventieth birthday, has always been the most active person I know. He skis, snowboards, plays basketball, kite boards, stand-up paddle boards, mountain bikes, hikes up mountains requiring an ice axe (!), and plays pickleball—you name it, he does it.

On the other hand, I played basketball and soccer in junior high and high school. But 99 percent of the time I would have preferred sitting and reading a good book than doing something exercise-related. On top of that, I was awkward, uncoordinated, and not very strong. I always had *potential* in the sports I played, but could never quite reach it. I blame part of that on my lack of confidence (I was a shy, self-conscious kid), and part of that on my total and complete lack of knowledge on how to get strong and fit. My older brother called me "Spaghetti Arms" throughout my teenage years and early twenties.

My arms were so weak I could barely even *hang* from a pull-up bar back then—let

1

alone do an actual pull-up. In those days, if you asked me to do a pull-up, I would have looked at you and said you were crazy—it wasn't ever going to happen.

So, it was a pretty unexpected turn in my life when I decided to get my personal training certification. At the time, I was living in Amsterdam with my husband, Brian, and I still wasn't very strong. I had managed to lose most of the freshman fifteen that I had gained in college, but a pull-up, L-sit, or even a few solid push-ups with good form was still out of the question for me. I diligently ran my three miles, three times a week (something I would never, ever do now because I equate slow running with torture), and experimented a little with lifting weights. But if you asked me to do a full push-up, a pistol squat, or even a bridge? I thought there was *no way* I'd ever be able to do it. I thought only freaks of nature could do those things, *real* athletes, and genetically gifted people who didn't happen to have long arms and an innate awkwardness.

But although I know now that my training in those days was less than effective, I still liked the changes I saw when I worked out consistently. I felt stronger, my clothes fit better, and my confidence soared. I was starting to appreciate exercise and how it could change people's lives for the better. Since I wasn't allowed to work in the Netherlands (I never was able to get a work visa), I took a leap of faith and decided to study for my personal training certification.

Fast-forward a couple of years later: I was working as a personal trainer in New York City, right near the East Village, one of my favorite spots in the entire city. I was working crazy hours as a trainer. I would get up at 5:00 a.m. to train clients, then be in the gym until 8:00 or 9:00 p.m. training the after-work crowd. On top of that, I was working out at least two hours a day on my own. I'd hop on the treadmill, then load up the barbells, do some isolation exercises like hamstring curls, triceps kickbacks, and calf raises, do even *more* cardio, and then keep lifting weights until my next client. Or until I was so tired I thought I might collapse.

During that time, I suffered constant, nagging, and usually weird injuries (a popped-out rib, a fractured foot, an immobile neck, among others). I was so exhausted and over-trained I had no energy left to do the things I really wanted to do, such as explore the city on foot with my dog, Rocket, go on a weekend bike ride with Brian, try new activities, or go hiking with friends. There was just simply nothing left after all the working out I was doing. On top of that, I was so hungry I was eating upward of four thousand calories a day (keep in mind I weighed about 140 pounds at the time). I wasn't fat by any means, but had trouble keeping lean. This was simply because I was exercising so much I just couldn't stop eating. I was always so hungry. It was a vicious cycle.

It was after one of those injuries that I started experimenting with HIIT and bodyweight training. I was sick of spending so much of my day stuck in a gym, and knew there had to be a more sustainable way to get—and stay—fit. My workouts went from two-plus hours a day to less than fifteen minutes most days. And as a natural result of the type of training I was doing, my equipment went from complicated machines and long waits at the gym to a few bars, a jump rope, and my own body.

The results shocked even me.

Not only did I have more energy, fewer injuries, and more time in my day—I also started getting leaner, stronger, and fitter than I had ever been (yes, even as a teenager)—and in an amazingly short amount of time. Before long, I was busting out pull-ups, triceps dips, and other exercises I'd previously thought were impossible. Since the workouts required so little space or equipment, I could do them in my tiny apartment using no equipment at all. Or head out to an outdoor fitness park with my jump rope and use the bars there, all while getting some fresh air. Best of all, I had a lot more time on my hands—time to do the things that I *really* wanted to be doing with my day, including, yes, reading a good book.

Soon after, I created 12 Minute Athlete to share the incredible benefits of HIIT and bodyweight training with the world. And now, after changing countless lives with the 12 Minute Athlete website and app, I am so excited to be sharing them with you here in this book.

Embrace the exercises and the workouts in this book and you *will* become fitter, faster, and stronger than ever before. But again, I can't force you to work out. It's up to you. Do you want to ditch your excuses and get in the best shape of your life? You decide.

WHY BODYWEIGHT TRAINING?

Most people think that the only way to get the fit and strong body they want is to work out with machines or heavy weights. *But most people are wrong.*

Because whether we like to admit it or not, the popularity of training equipment mostly comes down to marketing. Fitness companies need to have something to sell you, so they sell you machines, fancy gadgets, and complicated systems. So many of the new gadgets these companies come out with are utterly ridiculous. From the Shake Weight, a bulky, wobbly surfboard, to a bucking bronco (yes, this really exists), workout equipment just keeps getting weirder and more and more unnecessary. But unfortunately, when there are fit and attractive models demonstrating the equipment on TV, *somebody* is always going to buy it.

But training with your own bodyweight and just a few select pieces of equipment, like metal bars and a jump rope, is not only a more economical and less complicated way to work out, it will actually get you in incredible shape—unlike those mostly useless gimmicks.

And sure, barbells and a few pieces of uncomplicated equipment like dumbbells, kettlebells, and medicine balls can be useful tools to propel you to the fitness level you desire. But the truth is that you don't need *any* of these to get fitter.

Because the simplest and most effective way to develop strength, gain endurance, and lose fat is to train using nothing more than your own body.

Not convinced yet? Here's why bodyweight training should be a key component of your fitness regimen:

IT'S 100 PERCENT PORTABLE

What is the best thing about bodyweight training? You can do it anywhere.

It doesn't matter if all you have is a tiny studio apartment, a park, your parents' basement, or a hotel room—you can still work out. No excuses.

With bodyweight training, you don't need expensive gyms or fancy equipment. All you need is your own body, some motivation, and a tiny bit of space, and you can still get in a kick-ass workout, every single time.

IT USES YOUR ENTIRE BODY

When you train using your own bodyweight, most of the time you will be using all or nearly all the muscles in your body—rather than isolating just a few muscles at a time.

Why is this so great? For a number of reasons:

› Your body was built to work as a whole, so when you train using your entire body, you're ensuring you'll also be able to function well in real-life situations and daily activities.

› You burn more calories when you work all your muscles instead of just isolating one or two at a time.

› It turns your body into a fast-metabolizing, fat-burning machine.

› It leads to quicker and more noticeable results.

Pretty awesome, right?

IT BUILDS SUPER CORE STRENGTH

When machines got popular in the 1990s, people inevitably lost core strength. Why? Because when you're sitting down doing exercises such as biceps curls, shoulder presses, or lat pull-downs, you don't use your core very much—if at all.

On the other hand, when you do bodyweight exercises like push-ups, pull-ups, and squats, you are *forced* to use your core to maintain good form—meaning you'll end up having strong core muscles, without doing a single sit-up.

IT RESULTS IN FEWER INJURIES

When I constantly trained with heavy weights and machines, I would end up injured on a fairly regular basis. Whether it was shoulder issues from too many heavy overhead presses, a tweaked-out neck that couldn't turn to one side, or a rib that popped out of place (this does *not* feel good, trust me), heavy weights put us at a much greater risk of injury.

On the other hand, bodyweight exercises are much easier on your joints and less likely to put you at risk of overtraining. This also means you avoid accidents like dropping a barbell on your toe or smashing your finger between two weight plates.

IT MAKES YOU A BETTER ATHLETE

To be successful, most athletes need to be able to run, jump, and respond with incredible speed. They need stellar upper and lower body strength, as well as supreme balance and flexibility. They need to be able to use their body as a whole, not just in isolation.

Athletes need to constantly work at improving their fitness level to be the best they can be at their sport.

Since bodyweight training results in greater strength, power, endurance, speed, balance, coordination, and flexibility, it makes it the ideal method of training for athletes.

And if you use your own body as your gym, you'll become a better athlete, too.

LESS IS MORE

Forget about spending hours in the gym. Here's why shorter workouts are better than longer ones:

Shorter Workouts Make the Excuse "I Don't Have Time" Moot

When you know you'll be spending an hour or two working out, you are more likely to skip your workout altogether—which makes sense. An hour is a significant time commitment. You've likely got a million other things going on. But with short, intense, and minimal equipment workouts, that excuse goes out the window. *Everyone* has an extra twelve or fifteen minutes a day.

Don't agree? Just think about all the things you currently waste time on now: watching reality TV shows, taking really long showers, sleeping an extra fifteen or thirty minutes in the morning. No matter how busy your days are, you can easily shave off a few minutes here and there. You can definitely come up with enough time to get a twelve-minute workout in. Doing short, tough HIIT workouts makes it way more likely you'll actually stick to your workout schedule.

They Normalize Your Appetite

When you work out for hours on end, not only will your appetite grow to be enormous in order to make up for all the energy lost during your workout but you'll also put yourself at risk for that dangerous "I deserve this" mode—which can send your weight loss goals plummeting backward.

During my time as an in-person personal trainer, I can't tell you how many times I saw people do cardio and/or weights for an hour or more in the gym, and then immediately go across the street to Starbucks or Dunkin' Donuts and scarf down a giant-sized sugary drink and a pastry (or two!). All because they thought they worked hard, were ravenous, and felt they deserved a treat afterward. But sadly, this "reward" would nearly always result in a weight loss plateau, or worse, actual weight gain.

However, HIIT is different. Even though you have to work as hard as humanly possible during high-intensity interval training workouts, since you're not actually working out for a huge amount of time, you don't get that same "feed me now" feeling that you get after a really long run or weights session.

And science confirms it: Recent studies have shown that HIIT may actually suppress your appetite—while steady-state cardio can actually *increase* it. So train for shorter amounts of time. You'll likely feel less hungry overall.

They Show Results Faster

Need to get in shape quickly for the upcoming beach season, a high school reunion, or just to feel better and more confident about yourself? If you want to get the fastest results possible, don't go for a few steady jogs a week—do intervals instead.

HIIT has been in the press a lot lately, and for good reason. Recent studies have shown that HIIT can improve your fitness level in as little as two weeks, and can give you the same cardiovascular and muscular benefits as steady-state cardio in *half to one-third* the amount of time. Short but tough HIIT workouts, like the ones in this book, can also boost your metabolism, raise your body's fat burning power, and burn more calories in way less time.

They Get You in Better Shape in Less Time

I know there are people out there who actually *enjoy* long, steady cardio. But for the rest of us who dread spending hours feeling like a hamster on a wheel at the gym, knowing that shorter workouts are as (or more) effective than longer ones almost seems too good to be true.

"We now have more than ten years of data showing HIIT yields pretty much the exact same health and fitness benefits as long-term aerobic exercise, and in some groups or populations, it works better than traditional aerobic exercise," says Todd Astorino, a professor of kinesiology at California State University, San Marcos, who has published more than a dozen study papers on HIIT.

So get off the treadmill, and go do intervals. All your excuses just went out the window.

SHOULD MEN AND WOMEN TRAIN DIFFERENTLY?

I want to address something early on in this book because it's something that you probably have already noticed: I happen to be a woman.

When I first started in the fitness industry (almost a decade ago now), there were two styles of training: one for men and one for women. Unsurprisingly, workouts for guys were mainly focused on building muscle. And for women, it was all about getting skinny. Eight years later, I'm happy to say the industry has changed . . . a little. Men are still focused on building muscles and strength, but women are slowly becoming more okay with being fit and having visible muscles instead of striving for that malnourished look.

Yes! Progress.

Yet when it comes to actual fitness books, blogs, social media, etc., the worlds are still largely separate. Men write books for men. Women (and sometimes men) write books for women. But it doesn't have to (and shouldn't!) be that way.

When I first started 12 Minute Athlete in 2013, I consciously set out to create a training style that would work for both women *and* men. I wanted to bridge the gap between traditional men's workouts and women's workouts. I wanted to show that while yes, there may be some inherent differences between men and women, and certain things may come easier to one sex than the other, ultimately, both men and women are athletes—and they should train that way.

More than five years later, I'm happy to say that both girls *and* guys do 12 Minute Athlete workouts and get great results.

So, guys—don't think that the workouts in this book are "girly" just because they were created by a girl. They're not. In fact, I can't tell you the amount of times guys have told me they tried out a workout thinking it would be easy and ended up in a panting pile of sweat on the floor after only completing part of it.

And girls, don't think that the exercises in this book will make you look like a man— they won't.

Training with your own bodyweight will result in a lean, strong, and athletic body— for both women and men.

2.

BODY VS. MIND: WHY MIND-SET PLAYS SUCH AN IMPORTANT ROLE IN FITNESS

The process of setting a goal on the outer boundaries of what we think is possible, and then systematically pursuing it, is one of the most fulfilling parts about being human.

—BRAD STULBERG

GETTING YOUR MIND RIGHT AND SETTING EXPECTATIONS

Before starting the exercises and workouts in this book, let's first do a little mind-set work. While the physical work you put into the exercises is undoubtedly important, your mind-set going into these workouts will have a much bigger impact than you think.

If you go into the workouts and the program in this book absolutely 100 percent committed to getting stronger and fitter, you are going to come out stronger and fitter than ever before. You're going to completely level up your training, get stronger, master new skills, and prove to yourself just how awesome you really are.

On the other hand, if you half-ass your workouts, skip exercises you don't like, and don't give it your all, you're going to be disappointed with the results.

So, which will you choose? Are you all in?

SETTING EXPECTATIONS

If you commit to the workouts in this book and take advantage of all of the training resources I provide, you *will* get stronger and make progress on your goals. However, since everyone reading this book will naturally be at a different fitness level, it makes sense to set some expectations beforehand.

If you're starting from a more beginner or intermediate level of fitness, you will without a doubt see a ton of progress even in the first few weeks. That's one advantage of starting at a less advanced level—you have more room to grow. Just by consistency and repetition, you'll improve by leaps and bounds.

Keep in mind that building strength and new skills does take time. If you're starting out nowhere *near* doing a pistol squat or pull-up, you may or may not be able to do them within the next couple of months, but either way, you'll be well on your way to doing more advanced skills like these just by working the progressions. And if you diligently keep working on them, you *will* reach your goals.

On the other hand, if you're starting at a more advanced level, it's important to realize that since you don't have as far to go, your progress may be smaller. However, that doesn't mean you shouldn't expect progress at all—it will just be more of a fine-tuning at this level. For example, if you can already do a couple of pull-ups, by working the progressions and putting in the work you'll not only be able to do at least a few more; you'll also have better form and increased body awareness when doing them.

Wherever you're starting from, remember: I can give you all the best exercise progressions, workouts, and fitness tools in the world, but ultimately it's up to *you* to put in the work.

BUSTING THROUGH EXCUSES ONCE AND FOR ALL

Whether I'm traveling or at home in my beach town of Venice, California, I'm almost always working out outdoors. So when I'm doing a sweaty HIIT workout, busting out some pull-ups, or practicing handstands, I often get approached by a countless number of people. They'll usually say things like:

> › "If only I'd started ten years ago, I would be working out the way you do."
> › "I would *love* to be able to do [insert exercise here], but I work out at home and don't have a lot of equipment."
> › "If only I had more time to work out, I'd be trying to do what you do."

These excuses may be valid. But if you want to establish a lifelong workout habit, you need to recognize them for what they are: excuses. And no matter what your excuse is, there are a hundred ways around it. You just aren't seeing them yet.

FINDING A WAY AROUND YOUR EXCUSES

While it's easy to make excuses, excuses won't get you in shape. The good news is that finding a way to combat them isn't as hard as you might think—and once you begin to recognize them as excuses, you'll begin to train your brain to work around them.

To give you an idea of how to start doing this, here are some of the most common excuses and how you can bust through them:

YOU DON'T HAVE TIME

One of the most common excuses many people make is that they simply don't have the time, and if you think getting in a good workout means you have to spend an hour or two in the gym, no wonder you're not able to fit it in.

The key to working out consistently and still getting your workout done? Do shorter, more efficient workouts.

HIIT and bodyweight circuit workouts are as efficient as they come. You'll get more done in less time. You don't waste time sitting around resting in between exercises. The workouts will take you no more than twenty to thirty minutes to complete (including the warm-up), and you'll still have plenty of time to pursue your dreams, hang out with your friends and family, and do all the other things you need to (or want to!) do during your day.

YOU DON'T HAVE A GYM (OR MUCH EQUIPMENT)

Not having gym access is another major hurdle that stops people from exercising. Many people either don't want to spend the money for a membership or are intimidated by gyms, but you don't actually need a gym for a good workout.

Instead, consider purchasing a few good pieces of home workout equipment, such as a jump rope, a set of dumbbells, a sandbag, a medicine ball, and a pull-up bar. All are relatively inexpensive, easy to store, and will get you through years (if not more) of workouts.

If you really don't want to buy any equipment, there's also *so* much you can do using just your bodyweight. The workouts in this book, for example, are mostly equipment-free, and nearly every exercise that does use equipment has an equipment-free option.

YOU DON'T HAVE ANY ENERGY

We all get tired—and I'm certainly no exception.

But the funny thing about exercise is that the more you do it, the more energy you'll have. If you're someone who exercises regularly and then takes some time off from working out, you'll be surprised at how your energy levels will drop. There's just something about working out on a regular basis that actually makes you want to move even more—even outside your workouts.

So, the next time you're feeling tired, your muscles are a little sore or fatigued, or you're just plain not feeling motivated to work out, try seeing how it feels to work out anyway. Nine times out of ten, you'll not only feel more energized after your workout but you'll also be in a better mood, and be really glad you got yourself moving.

Keep in mind that there *are* legitimate reasons to skip a workout, including not getting enough sleep (aim for no less than seven to eight hours a night), being sick or injured, or even not eating enough that day. Learn to listen to your body and understand when a workout will reenergize it or when it's actually asking for a little extra rest. There's a fine line between regularly working hard and actually overtraining—which can hurt your performance and lead to greater fatigue, sickness, and a higher risk of injuries.

YOU'VE TRIED BEFORE WITHOUT RESULTS

Depending on your current level of fitness, it may take a few weeks, or even a month, to see and feel results from your workouts—no doubt a long time in today's instant-results society. Because of this, most people end up giving up too early and think they'll never be fit.

But it doesn't matter how many times you've tried before. If you work hard and stay consistent, you *will* get in shape. It's not going to be easy, but it will be worth it.

YOU'RE TOO OLD

Another one of the biggest excuses I hear from clients and readers is that they're too old to start working out or should have started when they were younger. Essentially, they're telling me that it's just too late for them.

But this is where I have to tell them that this line of thinking is complete BS.

I don't care how old you are. I don't care what your starting point is. I don't care if you didn't start exercising until you were forty-five or older.

No matter where you're starting from, you *can* make progress.

You've probably heard that you lose a small percentage of your muscle mass each year after the age of thirty. This is true—unless you do something to stop it. And yes, that *something* is resistance training. This can be with weights or your own bodyweight— either way, you'll be stopping that muscle decrease in its tracks. Not only can you put on muscle as you age but you can also get much stronger.

Later in this book, you'll encounter a ton of awesome exercises to help build your strength and a "bulletproof" body. Many of these exercises are very, very hard. You might look at them at first and think you'll never, ever be able to do them. But this is the wrong attitude to have.

What you'll notice is that I've also included a bunch of regressions for each of the exercises. Essentially, these are the baby steps that you'll use to build up the strength to do the more advanced version of the exercise. Stick with them, be patient, and you *will* get stronger and fitter—no matter where you are starting from.

FINDING YOUR "WHY"

Here's the thing: I can give you the very best fitness tools in the world, but if you don't actually *do* the hard work, you're not going to reach your goals. So how do you motivate yourself to exercise when there are dozens of things you'd rather be doing?

We all struggle with motivation at times (yes, even elite athletes don't *always* feel like training), so if you're not feeling particularly motivated every single day, you're certainly not alone. The key to creating both short- and long-term motivation is to find at least one (or ideally, several) intrinsic reason to keep going, even when you don't feel like it.

Intrinsic motivation means we do something because we are personally invested in the outcome. This is the exact opposite of extrinsic motivation, where we do things because we think we have to, or because other people tell us to. So how you do find your "why"? Here's how to start figuring it out.

FORGET (MOSTLY) ABOUT YOUR APPEARANCE

It's no secret that the majority of people exercise because they want to look a certain way or achieve a certain physique. But I'm going to tell you this right now: exercising for appearance's sake only is almost always a recipe for failure in the long run.

If you decide to work out and eat healthy *just* because you want to lose some weight, get a six-pack, or fit into a certain clothing size, every single thing you do that doesn't work toward that goal is going to make you feel like you're failing. Every dessert you decide to eat, every missed workout, and every rest day will most likely make you feel like you're sabotaging your goals. More often than not, this leads to an all-or-nothing mindset—meaning that at some point you're just going to give up altogether because you've already decided you're failing too often.

Sure, we all want to feel confident in our own bodies—and there's nothing wrong with wanting to look good. Just don't let it be your only, or main, motivation.

CREATING ATHLETIC AND SKILL GOALS

When clients and readers come to me with lackluster motivation, I always ask them one simple question: "What have you always wanted to be able to do?"

It usually takes a little prodding, but pretty soon I start to get answers like these:

> "I've always thought it would be *so* cool to be able to do a pull-up."

› "I've always wanted to compete in an obstacle race like a Tough Mudder."

› "I've always wanted to learn to do a back flip."

. . . and so on.

The answers are always varied, and sometimes they surprise me. But what I love the most is how every single person absolutely *lights up* when they tell me about their dream athletic or skill goals. *That* is your motivation. *That* is the reason you'll keep putting in the work every day, even when it's tough and the progress is slow. Because that feeling when you're finally able to do something you never, ever could do before . . . well, there's nothing quite like it.

Once you catch the athletic bug, it's often hard to stop. When I first decided I wanted to be able to do a freestanding handstand, my dream was to be able to hold a handstand without a wall for five whole seconds. Having no gymnastics background, five seconds seemed like a *huge* goal for me to achieve. Well, I worked hard at it, and eventually held that handstand for five seconds. But I wasn't content once I got there.

All of a sudden, I had dozens of new handstand-related goals. I wanted to be able to hold it for a minute at a time; to be able to move my legs in different positions while I was up there; to be able to press into a handstand, rather than simply kick up; to improve my overall line and efficiency; to be able to do a real one-arm handstand (aka not just a quick snap on Instagram where I put my hand up as fast as I can).

That first goal was just the starting point. From there, a whole new world of possibilities and additional goals opened up for me—and these goals have kept me endlessly motivated to put in the work.

CREATING ACTIVITY AND ADVENTURE GOALS

How many times have you caught yourself saying, "I've always wanted to [fill in the blank]"?

Whether that blank is to learn to kiteboard, to climb Mount Everest, to go surfing in Australia, to join an indoor soccer team, or to do something else entirely, most of us have activity and adventure goals that we'd love to actually do one day.

You also probably know that if you really want to take up a new activity or plan a new adventure, you'll need to reach a certain level of fitness first.

Yes, you'll need to *train* for your goals.

This is one of my favorite intrinsic motivations, because all of a sudden, no one is *forcing* you to work out or fuel your body with healthy foods. *You* start to want to train regularly so that you can do the thing you've always wanted to do. Your workouts begin to support your goals, and while you may not be hopping out of bed every morning eager to work out, you'll begin to be much more consistent and focused with your workouts. Why? Because you have a strong reason to do so.

IMPROVING YOUR DAY-TO-DAY LIFE

One side effect of training for performance instead of training for just appearance that most people don't consider is that getting stronger and learning to move your body better really improves the quality of your life, whereas dropping a few pounds probably won't affect it (unless we're talking about cases in which weight loss is necessary for medical reasons).

As you get stronger and forget about the scale, you become more likely to try to enjoy new sports and activities, play with your kids/nephews/nieces/siblings without getting tired, walk to the grocery store and carry your bags home instead of driving, lift your carry-on bag up on the plane yourself instead of asking for help, stay independent as you age, and so much more.

LONG-TERM HEALTH GOALS

Ultimately, you need to start thinking of health and fitness as a lifestyle, not a short-term habit.

If you're the type of person who has had times when you've worked out really hard for two months and then stopped completely for the rest of the year, this may be a complete reframing of your idea of exercise. But it's incredibly important.

Rather than thinking of working out as a temporary solution to lose weight, start viewing it as a long-term goal to live a longer and healthier life—one where you can keep up with your kids and grandkids, prevent many illnesses, and stay healthy and mobile into old age.

When you do that, working out becomes a privilege, not a chore—and there's no better motivator than that.

HOW TO SET MEANINGFUL GOALS YOU'LL ACTUALLY ACCOMPLISH

Without setting goals, you're much more likely to wander aimlessly through your workouts and your life. You'll miss out on so many ways you could be fulfilling your potential.

Yet in order to be effective, goal-setting *has* to go beyond a once-a-year scribbling down of New Year's resolutions. It's one thing to *have* goals and another thing to actually work toward them.

A couple of years back, I came across the book *The Art of Mental Training: A Guide to Performance Excellence* by D. C. Gonzalez while looking for books on sports psychology and mental toughness. I had been fascinated by the role of the mind in sports and other high-achieving endeavors for a while, and I really connected with Gonzalez's approach to achieving peak performance in sports, career, and life. The book also breaks down goal setting in the best way.

As Gonzales says, "Goals enhance performance and help create achievements."

Yet not all goal setting is created equal. Here's how to set meaningful goals you'll actually accomplish.

MAKE YOUR GOALS CHALLENGING—BUT REALISTIC

When you're setting your goals, make sure they're both challenging *and* realistic. Slightly out of reach goals are best because they require a lot of hard work, but they're ultimately still attainable with effort.

Some examples of goals like this would be doing your first pistol squat, competing in an obstacle race like a Tough Mudder, learning to do cool calisthenics moves like elbow levers, muscle-ups, or handstand push-ups . . . the list goes on. Even making a goal to audition for something as far-reaching as *American Ninja Warrior* is realistic for many people, no matter what level you're starting at.

On the other hand, a goal of going to the NBA when you're forty-five years old and have never played basketball before is not very realistic and probably isn't the best goal to set. Not that you can't *learn* to play basketball at this age—you just likely aren't going to go pro!

MAKE SURE THEY'RE *YOUR* GOALS

Think back to the Finding Your "Why" section on intrinsic motivation—don't create a goal to run a marathon just because everyone else is doing it. Figure out goals that excite you—whether it's to do your first handstand, climb Machu Picchu, learn to ski, or something entirely different.

Use your imagination. If you're not sure what your current goals are, you might need to think back to the things that interested you when you were younger. Even something as daring as skydiving at eighty years old is totally doable (yes, one *12-Minute Athlete* reader actually went skydiving for his eightieth birthday!). If it's something you've always wanted to do and you put your mind to it (and it's realistic), go for it. Ideally, your goals should both scare you a little *and* excite you.

STATE YOUR GOALS IN A POSITIVE WAY

When you're framing your goals, it's incredibly important to state them in a way that emphasizes what you actually *want* to happen, not what you want to *avoid* happening.

Why? Because our brains can really only hold on to one thought at a time, and when we state the negative—that is, "Don't choke toward the end of the game"—what do you think you'll end up doing? You guessed it—choking.

Instead, frame your goals in a positive way, such as "Play with confidence and to the best of my ability throughout the entire game," or "Shoot every free-throw in a calm and confident manner." This way, your brain can actually focus on what to do to get you to your goals, rather than dwelling on the negative. It makes a big difference—try it!

ATTACH THEM TO A TIMELINE

The worst thing you can do when creating goals is to have them be completely open-ended. For most people, this creates a scenario where they have a list of goals they wish to accomplish someday, but they never take a single step toward attaining them.

Instead, here's the method Gonzales lays out and the goal-setting method I've personally found most useful.

› START BY CREATING LONG-TERM GOALS. You can think of these goals as ones you'd like to accomplish in around one or two years (or more, but that's a good starting point).

› NEXT, BREAK YOUR GOALS DOWN INTO YEARLY GOALS. What would you need to accomplish in the next year to get you closer to your long-term goals? Try to be as specific as possible.

› FROM THERE, CREATE MONTHLY GOALS. This allows you to break down your goals even further and keeps you moving forward. For example, if your long-term goal is to be able to do ten pull-ups in a row, your monthly breakdown of this goal could specify how many days per week you want to focus on your pull-up training, what program or exercises you'll be following to help you get there, how often you plan on communicating with your accountability buddy, etc.

› LASTLY, CREATE DAILY GOALS TO HELP YOU REACH YOUR LONG-TERM GOALS. In the case of pull-ups, this would most likely just be your specific pull-up workout, post-workout journaling, stretching, and anything else you're doing that day to work toward your long-term pull-up goal.

DREAM BIG, ATHLETES!

Creating deliberate, well-thought-out goals will help you stay on track and accomplish way more in the long run. This method doesn't just apply to your fitness goals, either—I've personally applied it to career and life goals as well, with really great results. And don't forget, even if you don't accomplish a goal in a set amount of time, it doesn't mean *you* are a failure. We *all* fail, and failures can be some of the most valuable learning experiences—if we let them be.

After all, the only way to truly fail is to quit.

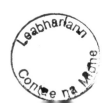

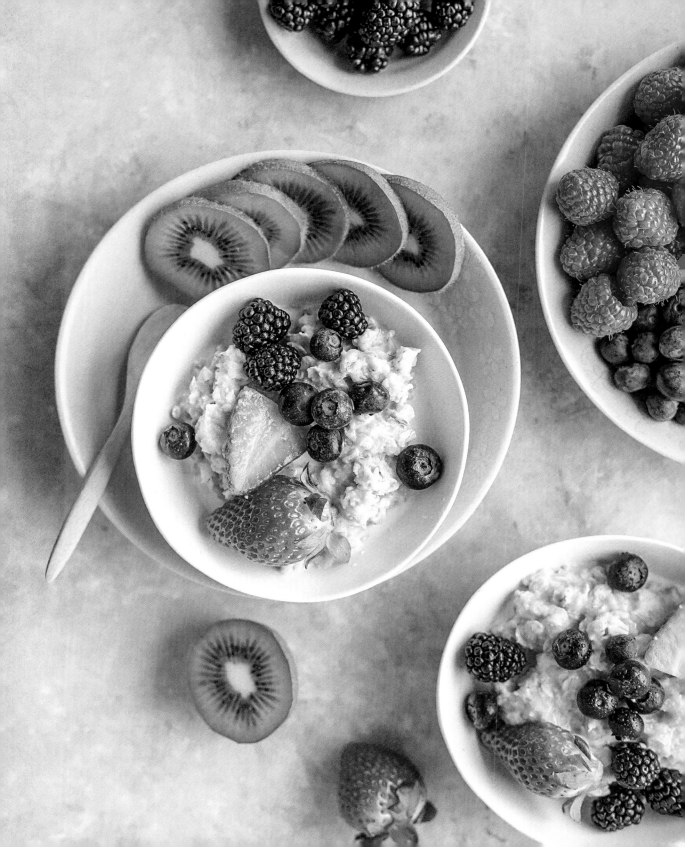

3.

FOOD IS FUEL: ADDRESSING THE ROLE OF NUTRITION IN YOUR WORKOUTS AND LIFE

Food is your body's fuel. Without fuel,
your body wants to shut down.

—KEN HILL

THE NON-DIET DIET: NINE NUTRITION RULES I SWEAR BY TO MAKE HEALTHY EATING EASY

Although this book is mostly focused on fitness, since that's my ultimate passion, there's no doubt that nutrition is an incredibly important part of your overall health and athletic performance. However, I'm not about to sell you on some new diet that's finally going to keep you lean, fit, and strong for life.

Why? Because diets suck. Not only do they leave you feeling hungry and deprived most of the time but they also make having any kind of social life nearly impossible, and make it more likely that you'll go on a binge-eating cheat-fest when your willpower inevitably weakens after a stressful day. Diets rarely work long-term. What's more, people who jump from diet to diet almost always tend to lose and then gain weight in a constant cycle. This yo-yo dieting, in turn, leads to feelings of failure, since it feels like nothing you do ever works.

Yet what you eat is an incredibly important piece of how fit and lean you are, so you can't ignore it completely. After all, abs are made in the kitchen. You can work out hard every single day, but if you don't eat well the majority of the time, you're not going to get the results you're looking for.

But eating healthy isn't as hard as you might think. Here are the nine nutrition rules I swear by to make healthy eating easy.

1. EAT AS MANY WHOLE FOODS AS POSSIBLE

Whole foods are any foods as close to their original state as possible. These will most often be foods from the produce aisle of your grocery store, and also include meats, fish, eggs, and grains like quinoa and brown rice.

Eating this way does require you to cook and prepare meals often, but it also leaves plenty of room for dining out at healthy restaurants.

2. INCLUDE PROTEIN IN EVERY SINGLE MEAL

Protein isn't just important for bodybuilders. We all should emphasize protein in our diets and try to include protein with every meal. Not only will getting in enough protein help keep you full longer but it will also help you maintain a lean and strong body—whether you're male or female.

It's also easier to do than you think. Just add in some extra egg whites to your eggs in the morning; Greek yogurt to your midmorning snack; or fish, chicken, or tempeh to your usual salad lunch. Most fairly active people or those looking to get leaner should aim for around one gram of protein per pound of bodyweight, or around 20–25 percent of your total daily calories.

If you're interested in learning more about sports nutrition and how your macronutrient intake can affect performance and fat levels, I highly recommend *Power Eating* by Susan Kleiner and any resources from Precision Nutrition.

3. EAT LOTS OF FRESH FRUITS AND VEGETABLES

This one may go without saying: fruit and vegetables are packed with nutrients that will help your body thrive and kick ass during your workouts and daily life.

Pile up your plate with veggies whenever possible—think kale, broccoli, cauliflower, Brussels sprouts, spinach, peppers, and whatever's in season. Don't like vegetables? You've probably just never had them cooked well. Get creative with your cooking style and bake them, steam them, grill them, or eat them raw in salads. You'll soon develop a taste for them and how they make your body feel.

Fruit is also an important part of your diet, but remember, you *can* eat too much fruit. Most active people should stick to two to four servings of fruit a day.

4. EAT PROTEIN AND CARBS AFTER EVERY SINGLE WORKOUT

After a really tough workout, your muscles need to repair. The best way to assist them? Eat a mix of protein and carbs as soon as you can after your workout—ideally within fifteen to thirty minutes, or at the most an hour.

A shake made with whey or vegan protein powder with frozen fruit is undoubtedly the easiest choice, but if you have more time you can also put together a meal like protein, rice, and veggies, or even protein pancakes (which are my favorite!).

5. EMBRACE FATS

No, I'm not encouraging you to gobble down handfuls of french fries. Healthy fats are where it's at. Think almonds, avocados, coconut, olives, and other healthy nuts and oils. You need more of these than you think!

Aim for healthy fats to make up 25–30 percent of your total daily calories.

6. EAT OFTEN

Eating less often and intermittent fasting are current trends in the health and fitness community, and they undoubtedly work for some people. Yet there's a reason that athletes traditionally eat more often (upward of five to eight meals a day): it works. Food is fuel for your body, and if you're doing intense workouts regularly and moving a lot throughout the day, eating smaller meals more often is your best bet.

Yes, I know this won't work for everyone. If you find that eating bigger meals less often works better for your lifestyle and your waistline, then by all means, keep eating that way.

7. DON'T AVOID CARBOHYDRATES

Low-carbohydrate diets may also be all the rage, but if you're looking to get stronger, build muscle, and become a better overall athlete, carbs need to be a consistent part of your diet. Not only do carbohydrates give you the energy you need to get through your workouts but they'll also help you recover faster and keep you energized and focused throughout the day.

Do your best to avoid refined carbohydrates and stick to quinoa, oatmeal, rice, and other nutrient-packed whole grains, as well as potatoes (sweet and regular) as much as possible. If you're fairly active, aim for about 50–60 percent of your total daily calories to be from carbohydrates. Less active people can consume less, but don't go too low or you'll feel the effects in both your workouts and your daily energy levels.

8. DON'T STARVE YOURSELF (EVEN IF YOU'RE TRYING TO LOSE WEIGHT)

Severely restricting your calories inevitably backfires in the long run, so don't do it. The key here is to remember that food is fuel. Give your body enough of the healthy food it craves. You'll be fitter, healthier, and happier because of it.

9. DON'T COMPLETELY DENY YOURSELF THE THINGS YOU LOVE

Love chocolate cake, cupcakes, or donuts? Fine, just don't eat them all the time. I advocate sticking to a healthy diet at least 80 percent of the time (more on this soon). This gives you plenty of room to cheat, to go on vacation, and to enjoy a happy hour with friends without feeling like you're a terrible failure as a person.

Food is wonderful and is meant to be enjoyed. Savor each meal!

For healthy recipes that will also satisfy your sweet tooth, like the homemade cashew cherry chunk energy bars shown on the next page, turn to the Recipes section in the back of the book; it begins on page 217.

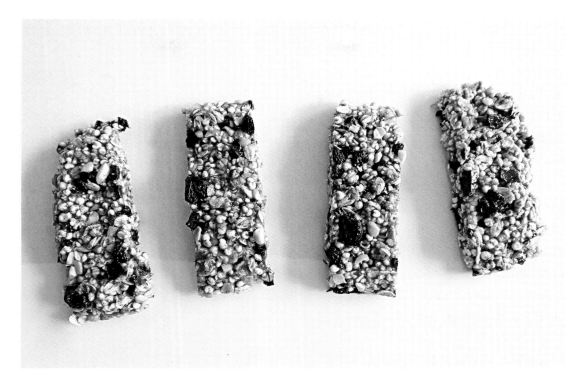

SEEKING BALANCE WITH THE 80/20 RULE

I stated before that you should try to eat healthy 80 percent of the time. But what exactly does this mean for your everyday eating?

IT MEANS THAT YOU DON'T HAVE TO COOK EVERY MEAL AT HOME

You know as well as I do that it's *way* easier to follow a 100 percent healthy diet when cooking your own meals. Cooking at home means you know *exactly* what goes into your food—how much oil, butter, how many carbs, etc. And it's about a thousand times easier to figure out your portion sizes.

That said, I like eating out—and I know I'm not alone here. I happen to be lucky enough to live in Los Angeles, a mecca for awesome restaurants and new places to check out. I like having other people cook for me as well, and I get a lot of joy out of finding new places to eat and exploring the city.

While I do try to cook my own meals the majority of the time, I typically eat out anywhere from five to seven times a week. Some of my meals out are similar to what I'd make at home—salads, veggie-packed stir fries, burrito bowls (I'm a huge fan of these as a healthy and filling meal when out and about). Some of them are also a little more indulgent—like trying out a great new pizza place, sharing Indian food with friends, or having a delicious, carb-loaded pasta or wood-fired oven pizza on a special occasion or as a Friday-night treat.

As long as I don't eat out too often, I don't feel guilty about these meals—and you shouldn't, either. Why work so hard in your workout if you're not going to enjoy and live your life?

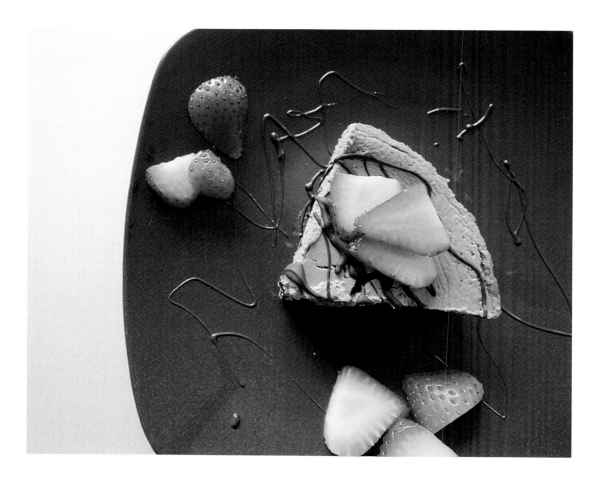

IT MEANS THAT ON BIRTHDAYS/HOLIDAYS/SPECIAL OCCASIONS YOU CAN HAVE A PIECE OF CAKE

One of the hardest things about trying to eat healthy is those big gatherings and events. Whether it's your nephew's birthday party, Thanksgiving dinner, or your best friend's wedding, it just feels wrong not to indulge a little—but when you do, it's also easy to feel like you are completely ruining your diet.

If you're living by the 80/20 principle, though, this way of thinking becomes completely unnecessary. Because as long as you're eating healthy most of the time and aren't out indulging in cake and sweet potato fries *too* often, you'll be totally fine.

I used to obsess over every single calorie at special occasions—even going so far as to avoid homemade pumpkin pie (my absolute favorite) at Thanksgiving, melt-in-your-mouth croissants in Paris, and homemade Christmas cookies around the holidays. I thought that if I did indulge, my entire diet would fall apart and I'd immediately gain twenty pounds.

Once I realized that was actually impossible, I started giving myself a little more flexibility in those situations—knowing that once the party/vacation/holiday was over, I'd naturally go back to eating healthily. I can't tell you how much happier and less bitter this has made me over the years.

IT MEANS YOU'RE BUILDING A LIFESTYLE, NOT JUST FOLLOWING A DIET

Most people who start diets inevitably fail. And it's true: most traditional diets just aren't sustainable long-term. They're based on restrictions and denying yourself your favorite foods 100 percent of the time. They're usually boring and unsatisfying, and more often than not, based on the latest fad decided by the health and fitness industry, usually with little long-term evidence to back them up.

What I want you to build, on the other hand, is a healthy lifestyle. I want you to start listening to your body, to realize that it actually craves protein, salads, and sweet potatoes most of the time. I want you to start relishing the taste of fresh strawberries, to experiment with new flavors and tastes, to order a kale salad instead of french fries at a restaurant not because you feel like you have to but because it just sounds better to your body.

If you give up dieting and focus on building a healthy lifestyle instead, you'll get there, sooner or later. Because as crazy as it might sound to you now, once your body starts getting used to eating adequate amounts of protein, fresh veggies, naturally sweet fruit; once it gets used to cutting out processed foods, not drinking soda, minimizing sugar; once you get used to feeling energized and pumped for your workouts; you won't want to go back. You'll feel better—and you'll want to start feeling that way all the time.

Then, when you have a cookie here and there, or a few too many chips at your favorite Mexican restaurant, it's just not a big deal. You'll enjoy every bite—but then you'll *want* to go back to your healthy meals.

It's all about allowing yourself little indulgences here and there, so you don't feel like you're depriving yourself of every type of food you've ever loved.

IT MEANS YOU DON'T HAVE TO BE PERFECT 100 PERCENT OF THE TIME

Nobody's perfect, and you might as well accept right now that you're not, either.

So, while it's a good idea to aim to eat healthy most of the time by not buying unhealthy foods, cooking at home when you can, and choosing wisely when you're eating out, you should expect to go off course at times.

In fact, allowing yourself a little give in your diet is actually a good thing. Because not only will eating perfectly 100 percent of the time make you feel bitter about life; it'll also make it more likely that you'll go on a binge-eating fest when your willpower is at its lowest. You'll end up chowing down on anything you can get your hands on.

Perfection is what leads people off course. It's what makes you down that entire bag of chips and pint of ice cream after a stressful day. It's because all you've eaten is boiled chicken and broccoli for a week straight, trying to be perfect.

Don't aim to be perfect. Aim to be *pretty good*, the majority of the time. That's the best you can hope for, and that's what's going to help you build a healthy lifestyle for the long run.

BALANCE IS KEY

In life and nutrition, it's all about finding balance. Because as much as you know that proper nutrition will get you the body you want, boost your athletic performance, and allow you to live a long, healthy, and active life, you also want to be able to just live a little. The 80/20 principle allows you to do that.

It's what allows you to go to a party and have something other than water, to be able to go to the new restaurant in your neighborhood and try the pizza everyone raves about, or to go to Paris and eat a croissant for breakfast instead of your usual protein shake or scrambled eggs.

It means you don't have to obsess about every morsel of food you eat. It allows you to try new things and be adventurous. Most of all, it gives you freedom—and that's what life is all about.

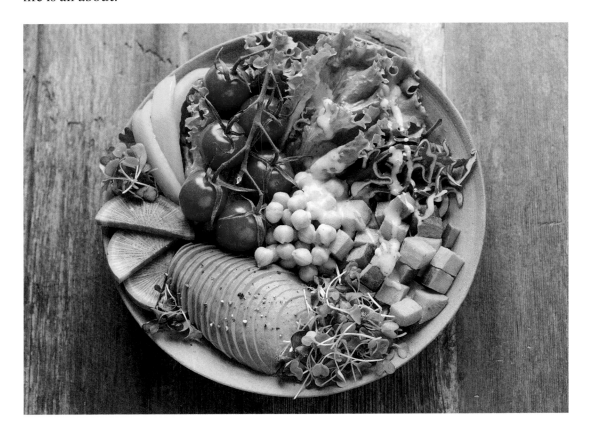

EATING FOR PERFORMANCE: PRE- AND POST-WORKOUT NUTRITION

How do you eat to perform well in your workouts? There's so much information about nutrition out there, it's really hard to decide what to believe.

I'm a huge fan of knowing your body and your individual needs, preferences, and of course, intolerances, if you have them. That way you can start to be critical when someone else tells you what exactly, and how much, you should be eating. Only you can figure out what works for your unique body!

That being said, one of the main principles I try to instill in my clients and readers is that *food is fuel*. If you go into a workout empty of fuel (calories), you'll most likely experience a crash partway through the workout, or at least not be able to work as hard as you would have if you'd eaten enough beforehand. Properly fueling up your body before a workout means that you'll be much more likely to crush it and set new personal records (PRs).

Similarly, refueling (that is, feeding) your body after a workout helps replenish your muscles so you can recover faster and be able to do your next workout sooner. As I mentioned before, since this book is mostly focused on fitness, I'm not going to go too in depth in this section, but it's important to know at least the basics of pre- and post-workout nutrition so that you can optimize your workouts.

WHAT (AND WHY) TO EAT BEFORE A WORKOUT

"What do I eat before working out?"

I get asked this question all the time. Because while most people know what to eat after a workout, they're clueless as to what they should be putting into their bodies beforehand. And the truth is, it's not an easy question.

Because like so many things in life, it depends on your own personal goals, and from my experience, there are basically three goals most people have when choosing what to eat before working out.

GOAL #1: EXTREME FAT LOSS

If your goal is to lose the maximum amount of fat possible, your best bet is to work out first thing in the morning without eating anything beforehand. Hence the term "fasted cardio," which you may or may not have seen thrown around in serious fitness blogs, magazines, and books.

Yes, you might feel dizzy, nauseous, or weak if you decide not to fuel up beforehand. And no, you won't be able to put in the full amount of effort you'd be able to put in if you worked out later in the day after eating a couple of good meals. But you will burn more fat.

GOAL #2: MAXIMUM PERFORMANCE

If you're looking to have the best workout possible and maximize performance, you won't skimp out on calories. You'll eat whatever it takes to fuel your body to help you perform the best you possibly can.

For example, if you are running a marathon, doing a triathlon, or competing in an important match or game, you wouldn't worry about eating too many calories beforehand. You're going for performance here, not weight loss. If that means a giant pasta dinner the night before, twice as much breakfast as you normally would eat, or downing sports drinks or energy gels during your race/event/game, so be it. Whatever you need to feed your body in order for it to do its best.

The drawback to this is that it's possible that you consume as many calories before (and after) your workout as you expend during your workout, making fat loss minimal to zero. In fact, some people even *gain* weight eating for maximum performance.

GOAL #3: FAT LOSS + PERFORMANCE

If you're like most people, most of the time your goal will be to lose fat or maintain your current leanness while still performing your best. What does this mean for you? It means you need to eat strategically before your workout. It does not, however, mean you should gorge yourself before your workout.

Whenever I've tried to work out without eating something beforehand, my performance suffers a lot. I get lightheaded and dizzy. I can't do as many reps. I just can't work as hard. Research backs this up, showing that exercise endurance improves significantly when you eat a snack beforehand.

So, assuming you're with me in boat #3 here, you should ideally be eating a full meal two to four hours before your workout, as well as a small snack thirty to sixty minutes before you train (this is optional and depends on your goals). The actual time may vary depending on how long it takes you to feel like you're not too full to work out. But don't wait too long after you eat or you'll realize you're hungry all over again (speaking from experience here).

WHAT—AND WHEN—TO EAT BEFORE A WORKOUT

So, what should a pre-workout meal consist of if your main goal is performance and fat loss? The ideal pre-workout meal should have some protein, some carbohydrates, and a little healthy fat. Yes, carbs! Carbs give you energy, and before and after your workout is the best time to consume them.

So again, it depends on your personal goals, but ideally you'll aim for something close to this:

> 10–20 grams of protein (this can be in the form of vegan or whey protein powder, dairy products like cheese or yogurt, or meat or a vegan substitute of your choice)

> 20–40 grams of slow-digesting carbohydrates such as oatmeal, sweet potatoes, beans, fruit, or wild rice (slow-digesting carbs produce a relatively slow increase in blood glucose and a modest insulin release in response)

> 5–10 grams of healthy fat (much more than this can slow down the digestion of protein)

Another thing to remember: the longer or harder your workout is, the more carbohydrates (and calories) you need beforehand.

PRE-WORKOUT MEAL IDEAS

Not sure how the above translates into an actual meal? Here are some pre-workout meal ideas to get you started:

› A PROTEIN SHAKE. Yep, you can have a shake before *and* after your workout. Aim for about 20 grams of fast-digesting whey or vegan protein powder and some carbohydrates from berries, oatmeal, or a banana, and a little nut butter or a scoop of flaxseeds to help keep you full.

› OATMEAL WITH FRUIT AND NUTS. Probably the perfect pre-workout meal, oatmeal with some nuts or a spoonful of your favorite nut butter mixed in and topped with your favorite fruit will give you both short- and long-term energy to power through your workout.

› VEGGIE OMELET WITH TOAST OR FRUIT. Eggs have both protein and fat and will keep you feeling full. The veggies and fruit will give you energy to push hard.

› PROTEIN OF YOUR CHOICE, SWEET POTATO, AND VEGGIES. The classic bodybuilder's meal (usually with chicken, but any protein will work), this takes a little more effort to cook, so the average person probably won't go for it—but it'll give you all the nutrients and energy you need to have a killer workout and build strong muscles.

› FRUIT, YOGURT OR COTTAGE CHEESE, AND LOW-SUGAR GRANOLA. Regular, Greek, or even coconut yogurt or cottage cheese is a quick and easy protein-packed choice for pre-workout snacking. Add some low-sugar granola and fruit and you'll be energized and ready to crush your workout.

› PROTEIN PANCAKES, BERRIES, AND A LITTLE NUT BUTTER. Protein pancakes are probably one of my favorite pre-workout meals, because they contain all the right ingredients and get me feeling pumped up for my workout. Just don't eat them too close to your workout since they're pretty filling and may leave you feeling queasy after only a few burpees.

Tip: To boost workout results even more, try downing caffeine an hour or so beforehand. Studies show that consuming 100–400 milligrams of caffeine before a workout in the form of coffee, green tea, or a pre-workout drink can boost energy and reduce fatigue during exercise.

Whatever you decide to eat before a workout, you'll probably need to experiment with what works for you and fits with your personal goals.

Do your best to listen to your body. Recognize the effects that food has on your performance—your energy levels, how soon you fatigue, whether you had any dizziness, stomachaches, cramps, etc. Then adjust as necessary to find the right pre-workout meal for you and your body.

POST-WORKOUT NUTRITION GUIDELINES

When you're working out, your body obviously uses energy. Carbohydrates are the first macronutrients that your body uses for energy. They are stored in your muscles as glycogen, so after a hard workout, your glycogen storages are pretty empty. It's super important to refill them to get the recovery process going.

As the building block for our muscles, protein is also a crucial component of a post-workout meal. Protein rich foods are also very filling. Think about eating a post-workout meal like you were building a house: to build a strong and beautiful house, you need high-quality materials, so make sure to refuel with high-quality food after your workout! It will help you build a strong and powerful body.

IS A POST-WORKOUT MEAL ABSOLUTELY NECESSARY?

In general, it's recommended to eat as soon as possible after your workout, preferably within thirty minutes. However, there are some things worth asking.

DID YOU WORK OUT FASTED OR FUELED?

If you're working out fasted (that is, you haven't eaten for eight or more hours), it's generally very important to eat a post-workout meal as soon as possible, preferably within fifteen to thirty minutes after training.

If you've had some food within a couple of hours of your workout, your glycogen stores are probably not exactly depleted. Don't be too concerned if you can't or simply don't want to eat right after your workout, especially if your workout was lighter, involving something like moderately paced cardio or yoga.

HOW INTENSE WAS THE WORKOUT?

If you just did a HIIT or a tough bodyweight workout and totally depleted your energy levels, then the sooner you eat your post-workout meal, the better. The same is true for other workouts that burn a lot of energy. For example, if you go for an hour-long run, you'll also burn a lot of energy, so you need to refuel as soon as you can afterward to promote optimum recovery. If your workout was something relatively light that didn't demand a lot of energy, there's no need to eat right away. Feel free to eat later when you get hungry.

The problem with "mandatory" post-workout eating is that people who didn't actually use a whole lot of energy (or ate a big pre-workout meal) think that they need to eat a proper, often high-calorie meal immediately afterward. That may easily lead to overeating, because these people are overestimating the caloric expenditure from a workout and the amount of food that they actually need. Healthy foods also add up and instead of helping to lean out and gain muscle, the excess calories get stored as fat.

THE IMPORTANCE OF A POST-WORKOUT MEAL AFTER A HIGH-INTENSITY WORKOUT

Since most of you reading this will likely be working out like athletes and burning a lot of energy during your workouts, it's critical to replenish the energy you used during your workout as soon as you can. Refueling after a high-intensity workout is important for two reasons that are closely related:

›   FASTER RECOVERY. You want to recover from your workouts as fast as you can. You want to not only feel less sore and fatigued but also ready to work out again as soon as possible so you can keep working toward your goals. If you don't provide your body with quality energy (aka food) soon after your last workout, you'll most likely end up tired, fatigued, and sore. You definitely won't feel ready to work hard during your next training session.

›   MUSCLE BUILDING. Muscle growth is possible only if you eat enough.

That's especially true after your workout when your muscles are ready to put all the nutrients that you give them to good use. Eating a good balance of protein and carbs post-workout will help you achieve leanness and muscle growth.

During hard workouts, you cause micro tears in your muscles. To help them heal (which in turn leads to faster recovery and muscle building), make sure to eat a good post-workout snack or meal after each tough workout.

MACROS IN YOUR POST-WORKOUT MEAL

The most important thing about post-workout meals is that they should include both carbohydrates and protein. If you don't feel like having a full meal right after working out, at least have a snack like a protein shake soon after—then you can have a full meal later on.

For optimal muscle recovery after a hard HIIT or bodyweight workout, aim for an approximately 3:1 carbs-to-protein ratio.

Here are some examples of good carb and protein sources that you can combine into a balanced post-workout snack. You can mix and match these foods, choosing one carb and one protein rich food.

If you use these amounts, the carbs-to-protein ratio will be approximately 3:1 (not all combinations give you exactly this ratio, though; if you choose higher carbs, also choose higher protein). Research shows this ratio is the most appropriate for ultimate muscle recovery.

CARB SOURCES:
  › ½ cup oats (150 kcal / 27 g carbs)
  › 1 medium-sized banana (105 kcal / 27 g carbs)
  › 1 medium-sized cooked sweet potato (103 kcal / 24 g carbs)
  › 3 tbsp raisins (99 kcal / 24 g carbs)
  › 1 cup blueberries (84 kcal / 22 g carbs)

PROTEIN SOURCES:

> › ¼ cup canned tuna (50 kcal / 11 g protein)
> › ¼ cup chicken breast (52 kcal / 10 g protein)
> › String cheese, 1 stick (80 kcal / 7 g protein on average)
> › ¼ cup cottage cheese (45 kcal / 7 g protein on average)
> › 1 hard-boiled egg (70 kcal / 6.5 g protein)
> › 1 serving tofu or tempeh (95 kcal / 10 g protein on average)
> › 1 serving whey or vegan protein powder (120 kcal / 20g protein on average)

When you pair one carb and one protein food from this list, your snack will end up being around 200–300 kcal.

To make larger meals, simply adjust the portion size so that you're consuming bigger portions of the same foods with similar ratios. Add in some veggies, and you have a healthy, nutrient-packed meal that will support your recovery and get you back to training in no time.

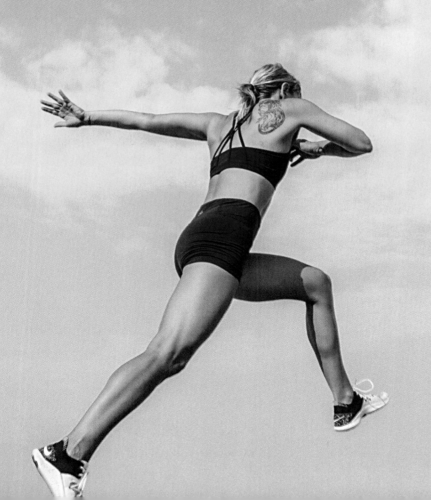

4.

BUILDING SUPERHUMAN STRENGTH WITH BODYWEIGHT EXERCISES

Strength doesn't come from what you can do.
It comes from overcoming the things
you once thought you couldn't.

—RIKKI ROGERS

The exercises in the next few chapters will get you stronger and in better shape than you ever thought possible. Best of all, they require very little equipment—or time—to complete.

Follow the progressions in these pages and you'll build superhuman levels of strength and endurance like never before.

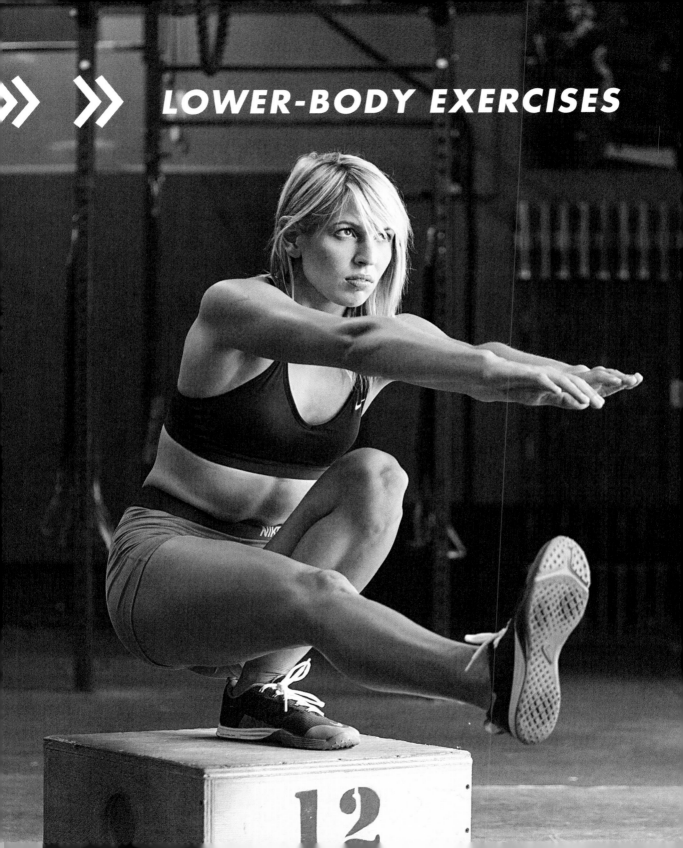

SQUATS FOR A STRONG LOWER BODY

Not only will squats give you a strong lower body and make you look good but they'll also improve your overall athleticism and make you a better, more functional, and well-rounded athlete overall. And although weighted and barbell squats certainly have their purpose, you should never discount the awesomeness of the simple bodyweight squat, also known as an air squat.

Here are just a few reasons to master the bodyweight squat:

› BODYWEIGHT SQUATS ARE 100 PERCENT PORTABLE. You can do them anywhere, anytime!

› THEY'RE SILENT AND TAKE UP PRETTY MUCH ZERO SPACE. If you need to be quiet or simply don't have much space, you can still do bodyweight squats.

› THEY ENGAGE YOUR ENTIRE BODY. If you do air squats right, not only will they strengthen your legs and butt muscles but they'll also work your core.

› THEY INCREASE MOBILITY. To be able to squat properly, you need basic hip, ankle, and torso control. Working on your squat will increase mobility and flexibility in each of these joints, and make you less prone to injury.

› THEY'RE THE PERFECT EXAMPLE OF FUNCTIONAL FITNESS. We squat every day in our normal lives, and adding them to your workouts makes it less likely you'll get tired and injured in everyday activities.

› EVEN THOUGH YOU'RE NOT USING WEIGHTS, AIR SQUATS WILL STILL MAKE YOU SUPER STRONG. Do twenty, or forty, or a hundred, and you'll feel it, I promise.

HOW TO DO BODYWEIGHT SQUATS

Although they may seem like a basic human movement, unfortunately, due to improper training, lack of strength, and/or mobility and flexibility, most people don't do air squats properly—which is a recipe for injury or creating an unbalanced body.

Here's how to do them correctly:

›   Stand with your feet about hip-width apart, with your toes pointed forward or slightly outward. Your arms should be hanging relaxed by your side. Engage your core muscles and push out your chest slightly by pulling your shoulder blades toward each other.

›   Bend your knees and push your butt and your hips out and down behind you as if you were sitting into a chair. Keep your weight on your heels.

›   Squat down until your thighs are below parallel to the ground, or as far down as you can get them. Eventually, you'll want to work up to getting your butt sitting on the back of your calves, but if you're not there yet, don't worry—you'll get there with time and practice. As you lower down, you can choose to raise your arms in front of you or keep them by your side. Try to keep your chest upright with your shoulders pulled back.

›   As you stand back up, straighten your legs and think about squeezing your glutes and keeping your knees externally rotated. (Think about pushing your knees out; don't let them turn inward.)

BODYWEIGHT SQUAT KEY POINTS

•   Keep your weight on your heels.

•   Keep your torso upright with your shoulders pulled back.

•   Your feet should be hip-width apart with your toes pointing forward or slightly outward.

•   Your glutes, upper back, and core muscles should be engaged.

•   On the downward portion of the squat, you should aim to go below parallel.

•   On the upward portion of the squat, keep your torso upright, push your knees out, and squeeze your butt. It may help to bring your arms in front of you as you stand up.

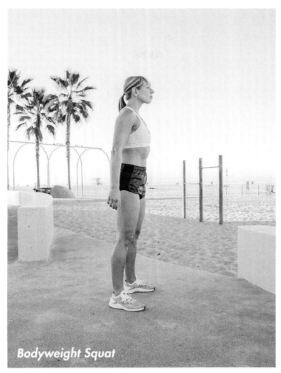

Bodyweight Squat

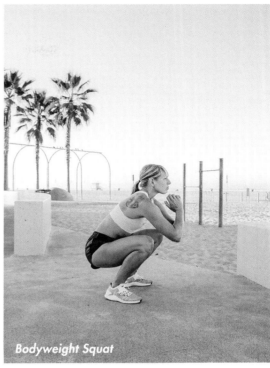

Bodyweight Squat

PISTOL SQUATS: THE ULTIMATE BODYWEIGHT LEG EXERCISE

Arguably the very best lower body exercise of all time, pistol squats require incredible leg strength, flexibility, and balance. If you've never tried them before, I'll warn you: pistol squats are *tough*.

But here's the thing: if you think you could never do a pistol squat, think again. Because if you follow the progression of exercises below, before you know it, you'll have built the necessary strength to master the ultimate leg exercise.

Start wherever is most appropriate for your current strength and flexibility level—that is, there's no need to start at the beginning if you can easily do a one-legged bench squat already (although working on this will still help you build up strength). Then make sure to include these exercises in your workout routine two to four times a week for the fastest possible results.

So, whether you're starting from zero and have never done a pistol squat in your life or you can do a few right now and want to be able to do more, here's how to begin mastering pistol squats:

BOTTOM OF PISTOL HOLDS

Believe it or not, the bottom position of the pistol squat is actually the hardest part of the exercise for a lot of people. Holding the bottom position will help you to build up strength in your core and hip flexors, as well as develop the muscle memory for the correct movement of the pistol squat.

› Squat down into a full deep squat with your glutes sitting on the back of your calves.

› Extend one leg in front of you, engage your core, and try to straighten your extended leg as much as possible.

› Hold this position for time.

› If you need to hold on to something for balance to start, that's fine.

Work up to holding the bottom of pistol position for three rounds of thirty-second holds.

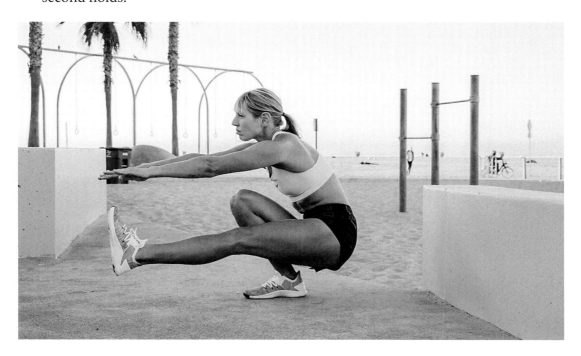

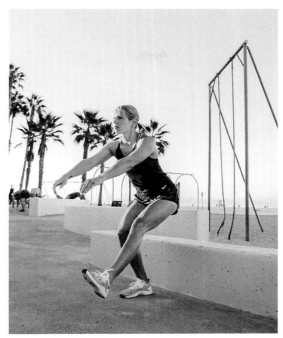 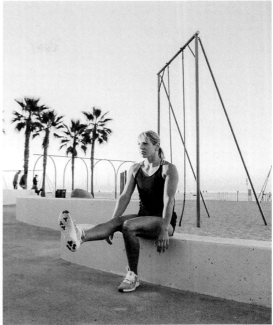

ONE-LEGGED BENCH SQUATS

One-legged bench squats will help you build up the strength to do pistol squats as well as help your body understand the correct feeling of the movement.

> Stand in front of a bench or a sturdy surface (the higher the surface, the easier this exercise will be).

> Straighten your opposite leg out in front of you, push your hips back, and sit down, keeping your leg as straight as possible. It's okay if you fall down the first few times: keep working at it and you'll gain control with practice. Go ahead and hold on to something for support if you need to.

> Engage your core, squeeze your butt, and pull your shoulders back as you try to stand back up.

If you need assistance from this position, lightly rest the heel of your lifted foot on the ground and use it to help you balance as you stand up. As you get stronger, try doing this on lower surfaces to continue to challenge yourself. The lower the surface, the harder this exercise will be.

Work up to three rounds of eight one-legged bench squats per leg.

ASSISTED PISTOL SQUATS

Once you're feeling comfortable doing one-legged bench squats at knee height or lower, you can start working on assisted pistols. These will help you get the movement of a pistol down, while not requiring the strength needed to do the full thing.

› Hold on to a sturdy object like a pole or a door frame and lower yourself down to the bottom position of the pistol squat with as much control as possible.

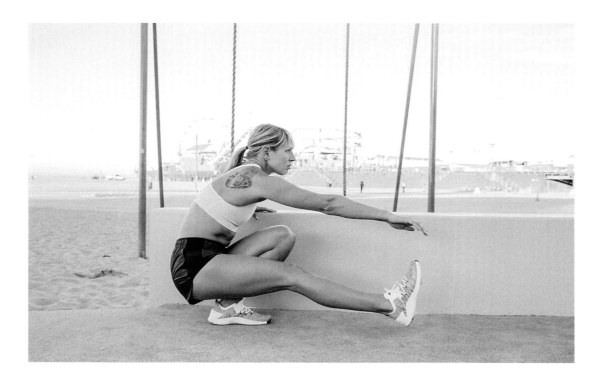

> Relying as little as possible on your arms to help you get back up, push your hips back, engage your core, and stand up.

You can also use bands or a TRX for a similar effect (helpful if you don't have anything sturdy to hold on to).

Work up to three rounds of five assisted pistol squats per leg.

ELEVATED PISTOL SQUATS

One of the hardest parts about a pistol squat for most people is that along with needing really strong legs to be able to squat on one leg, you also need to keep the other leg straight in front of you, which requires not only a ton of strength, but also balance and flexibility. Elevated pistols can help you work up to building the strength and muscle memory you need for a full pistol squat, since your leg doesn't have to remain as straight when doing them.

> Find a sturdy elevated surface such as a bench or a box and stand on top of it.

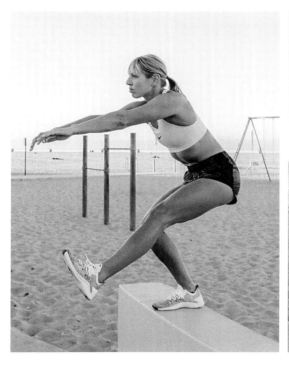
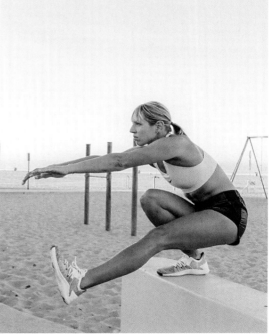

› With your arms extended in front of you, stand on one leg, keeping your opposite leg extended as straight as possible.

› Push your hips back, lean forward slightly, and raise yourself back up to the starting position. If your opposite leg dips below the bench, that's okay—keep practicing!

If you need to, you can start out by holding on to something close to you such as a pole, doorway, or even putting your hand on a wall to assist yourself. Then work up to doing these without holding on to anything.

Work up to three rounds of five elevated pistols per leg.

NEGATIVE PISTOL SQUATS

Negative pistol squats help you get used to the movement of pistols and increase your strength.

› Hold your arms out in front of you, then stand on one leg with your free leg held straight out in front.

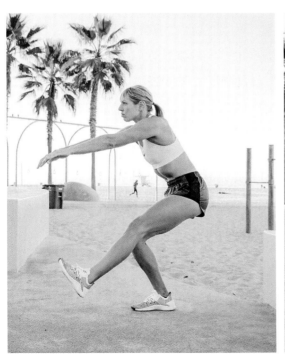
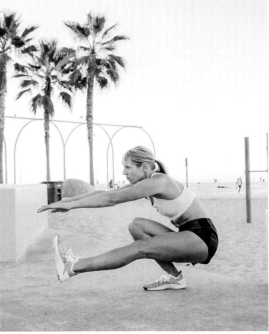

> Push your hips back and slowly lower down so that your butt is almost touching the ground. *Really* fight to lower down as slowly as possible— aim to take ten seconds or longer for each negative rep.
> Set your other leg down, then stand back up with two legs.

Work up to three rounds of five negatives per leg.

FULL PISTOL SQUATS

Ready to try the full thing? Awesome! You're a badass, even for just trying it.

> To do a pistol squat, start by holding your arms out in front of you, then stand on one leg with your free leg extended straight out. Push your hips back and sit down as far as you can so that your butt is almost touching the ground. It's fine if you need to lean forward slightly to get in the right position.
> Once you hit the bottom position, pause briefly, then engage your core and squeeze your glutes as you stand back up on one leg.

As you get better at doing full pistol squats, continue to refine your form and work to reduce any momentum on the way up. A great goal to work toward is three rounds of five solid pistols per leg.

Full, unassisted pistols are not easy. If you can do them, or get anywhere close to doing them, you should be proud of how strong you've become!

TROUBLESHOOTING PISTOL SQUATS

If you're having trouble with a specific aspect of the pistol squat, the exercises that follow will help. Remember to be patient with your progress— depending on where you're starting from, working up to a full pistol squat on each leg may take time. The most important thing is that you work your pistols consistently and don't give up.

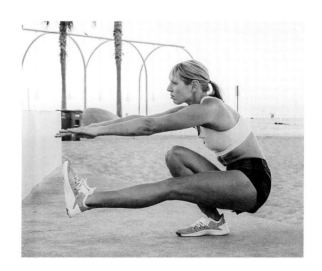

CANDLESTICK PISTOL ROLLS

Adding in momentum can help some people achieve a pistol squat faster than focusing on the other progressions.

› From standing, squat down, roll onto your back, and lift your legs straight above you in a candlestick position. Try to keep your knees as straight as possible and your toes pointed as you engage your core.

› Bend one knee as you quickly lower it to the ground touching or almost touching your butt. Use momentum from the roll and lean forward and stand up as you keep your other leg as straight as possible.

› Immediately jump into the air on one leg with your arms above your head, then repeat on the other side. Try to minimize the amount you use your hands to help you up.

Beginner variation: To make this exercise easier, roll back on an elevated surface such as a raised mat or couch, or simply stand up with two legs instead of one.

Work up to doing three rounds of five candlestick pistol rolls per leg.

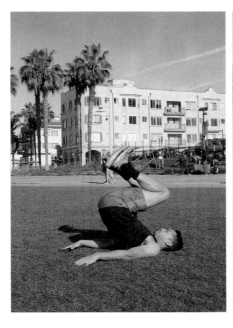 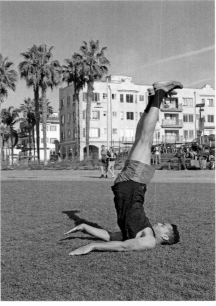

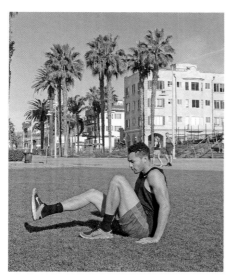
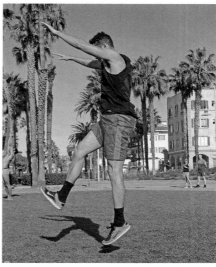

HIP FLEXOR TRIANGLES

If you're having trouble holding your leg up at the bottom of the pistol squat, it's most likely due to weak hip flexors. Hip flexor triangles work wonders to increase hip flexor strength.

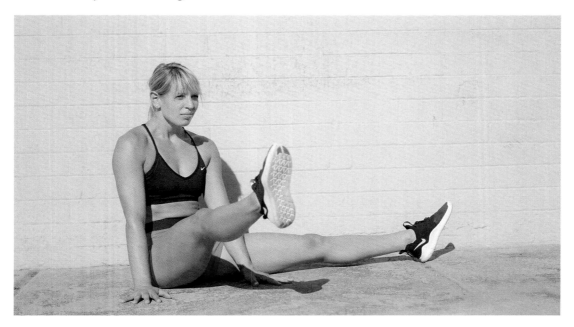

> Sit on the ground with your legs straight in a straddle position and your hands on the floor in front of you.

> Keeping your leg as straight as possible, raise one leg off the ground and bring it as high as you can toward the midline of your body.

> Lower your leg down in front of you without actually touching the floor, then bring it back to the starting position. That's one rep.

Work up to doing three sets of ten to fifteen hip flexor triangles per leg.

OTHER TROUBLESHOOTING METHODS

> USE COUNTERWEIGHTS. Pistols are one of the only exercises where holding out a weight in front of you can make the exercise easier. Try holding anywhere between five and ten pounds straight out in front of you at chest level to help you work up to full pistol squats.

> PARTNER PISTOLS. Grab on to a partner's hands so that both of your arms are straight out in front of you. The two of you should lower down at the same time, then use each other's weight to help each other to push past the sticking point on your way up.

ADDITIONAL LOWER-BODY STRENGTHENING EXERCISES

Although you can certainly focus only on basic bodyweight squats and pistols and build strong, powerful legs, there will undoubtedly be times when you'll want to switch up your leg workouts to build additional strength, push past a plateau, or just do something different for a change.

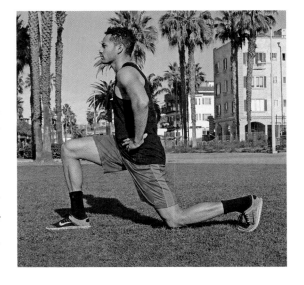

The following exercises are all fantastic options for strengthening your lower body. And although every single one of these exercises can be done using only your own bodyweight, you can also make them more challenging by adding weights of any sort—a sandbag, kettlebell, or simply a backpack filled with heavy stuff are all perfectly acceptable options.

BACK LUNGES

› From standing, step one leg back behind you in a lunge position.

› Keep your core tight and your torso upright as you return to standing.

BULGARIAN SPLIT SQUATS

› Stand in a split stance with your leg elevated on a box, bench, or raised surface behind you.

› Keep your front foot on the ground, engage your core, and pull your shoulders back, then bend your knees until your back knee is close to the ground.

› Squeeze your glutes and keep your core engaged as you stand back up. Repeat on both sides.

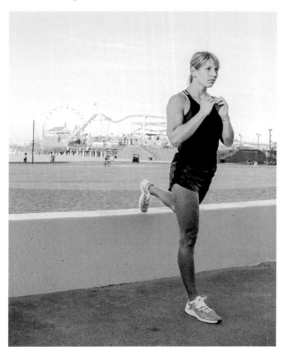
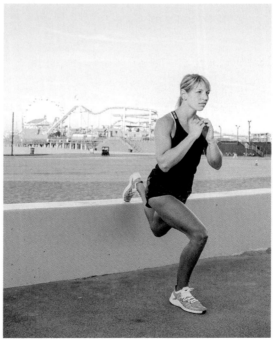

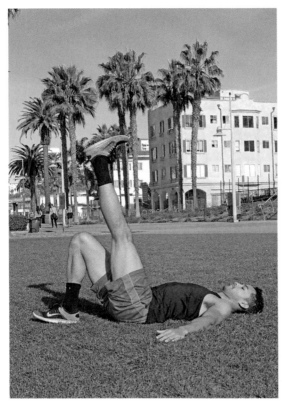 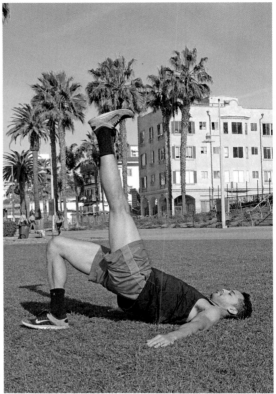

CANDLESTICK HIP BRIDGES

›   Lie down on your back with your knees bent and feet on the floor.

›   Raise one leg up straight above you, engage your core, then lift your hips up as high as you can while you squeeze your glutes.

›   Lower down with control, making sure to work both sides.

SIDE LUNGES

›   Stand with your legs wider than hip-width apart so that you're in a standing straddle position. The longer your legs, the wider you'll need to stand.

›   Lean toward your left leg, bending down as far as possible while keeping your core engaged and chest up.

› Eventually, your goal will be to get your hamstring (the back of your leg) to touch your calf, but don't worry if you're not there yet.

› Squeeze your glutes as you stand back up, then lean toward the right leg. Try to keep your torso upright and core engaged the entire time.

If you're having trouble balancing with this exercise, hold on to a sturdy surface in front of you like a chair or a bench (a band or a TRX also works) to help you build the muscle memory for the movement.

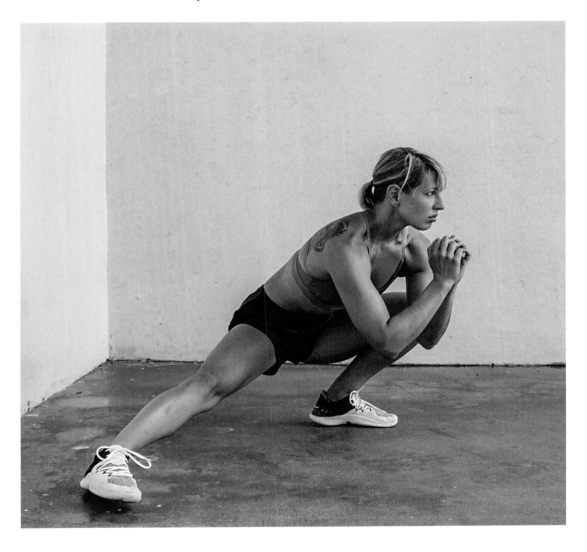

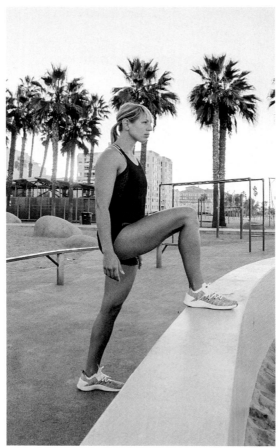 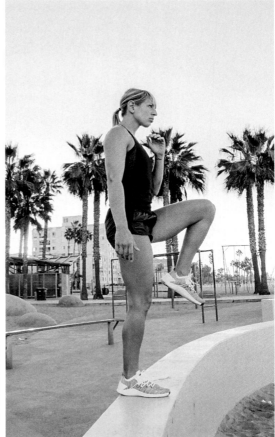

STEP-UPS

> Stand in front of a plyo box, bench, or sturdy elevated surface, then step up first with one leg onto the platform, immediately following with your other leg.

> Squeeze your glutes and keep your core pulled in tight.

> Your legs should be straight or slightly bent at the top position.

> Step back down, then lead with your right leg.

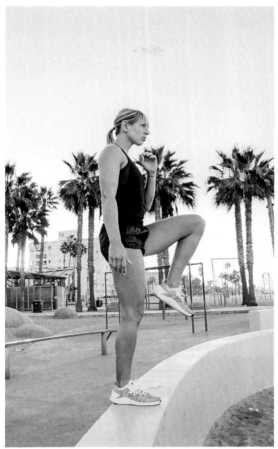 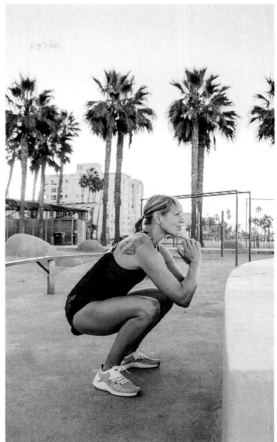

SQUAT STEP-UPS

› Stand in front of a plyo box, bench, or elevated surface.

› Step up onto the surface with one leg, following with the other leg.

› Step back down, then immediately squat down.

› Repeat starting with the other leg.

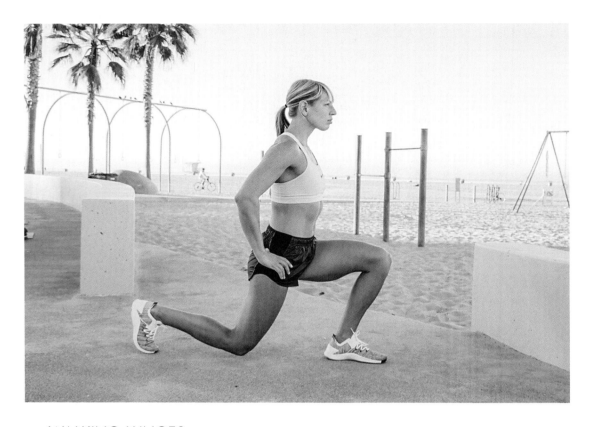

WALKING LUNGES

› Start in a lunge position with your back knee touching or almost touching the floor (if you're doing these on a hard surface like concrete, please don't smash your knees into the ground!).

› Without pausing, alternate legs, bringing your opposite leg forward into a lunge position.

› Think about keeping your chest up and shoulders pulled back while you continue alternating legs and moving forward.

PLYOMETRIC LOWER-BODY EXERCISES

See the section on plyometric lower-body exercises on page 146.

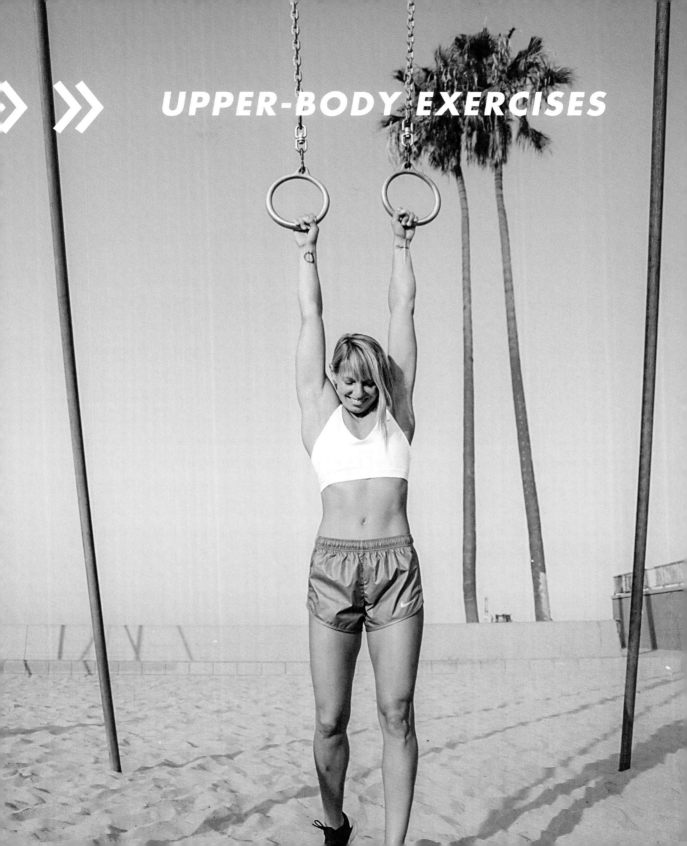

PULL-UPS: RELEASE YOUR INNER BADASS

I know what some of you must be thinking: I can't do a pull-up, and unless I spontaneously turn into a superhero someday, I never will.

But the truth is, if you're one of the majority of people who can't currently do a pull-up, it's probably more of a mental issue than a strength one. Or, at least, that's the long-term reason you can't do a pull-up, since strength may indeed be stopping you from doing one in the short term.

Many people, especially women, assume they won't ever be able to do a pull-up. As in, they truly believe it's physically impossible. In fact, even the *New York Times* claims that women—and men of a certain stature—can't do pull-ups. Back in 2012, the newspaper published an article titled, "Why Women Can't Do Pull-ups," that pissed a lot of people off (including me). Even worse, it made those people who can't currently do pull-ups believe even more strongly that they will never be able to do even one.

Basically, the article noted a study where exercise researchers from the University of Dayton found seventeen women who couldn't do a single overhand pull-up and put them on a weight-lifting routine for three months. They then gave them exercises to do three days a week aimed at strengthening their arm and back muscles. When, by the end of the three-month time, only four of the women succeeded in doing a pull-up, the researchers basically concluded that women (and certain men, notably those who were taller and with longer arms) weren't suited to do pull-ups because of their stature and/or higher body fat percentage.

But whether you're male or female, young or old, athletic or a workout newbie, you shouldn't accept that you can't do a pull-up just because the *New York Times* tells you that you can't.

Because here's the thing: it takes *time* to build up the strength necessary to do pull-ups and other tough calisthenic exercises. Elite gymnasts work for *years* to build strength and perfect their movements—why should the average, non-elite athlete expect to build strength more quickly?

More likely than not, the women in the study simply weren't given enough time or the right exercise progressions to gain the proper strength to do pull-ups. If you've never done a pull-up in your life, you're not going to be able to do one in two weeks. But take the time to build up a solid foundation and you'll be busting out pull-ups into old age.

WHY YOU SHOULD LEARN TO LOVE PULL-UPS

Without question, pull-ups are the ultimate badass upper-body exercise. In fact, they're probably my very favorite bodyweight exercise of all time—and I know I'm not alone here.

Yet for most of my life, I was just like many of you: unable to do a single pull-up. Heck, I couldn't even do a push-up. But of course, like most pull-up nay-sayers, I never even tried more than a halfhearted attempt at an assisted pull-up once every couple of years or so. Of course I sucked at pull-ups—it's easy to see that now.

So, if you still think you'll never be able to do a pull-up, think again—because if you follow the progression of exercises described in this chapter, you'll build the strength necessary to be able to do one, two, maybe even ten or twenty pull-ups. Once you've got those down, you can move on to even cooler exercises like one arm pull-ups and muscle-ups. But in order to get strong enough to do those more advanced exercises, you need to build up your foundation first.

So that's where you're headed next. You're going to build up your foundation so you can be the ultimate pull-up master, build a strong upper body, and impress the hell out of your friends.

FLEX HANGS

When you're first starting out with pull-ups, you need to start building up strength in your back, arms, and core, as well as strengthening your grip, and flex hangs are the best way to do that.

› Use a bench or a chair to boost your chest up to the pull-up bar, and then simply try to stay up.
› You'll probably want to start out with your hands in an underhand (chin-up) grip, but work on switching to an overhand grip as well once you get comfortable enough.

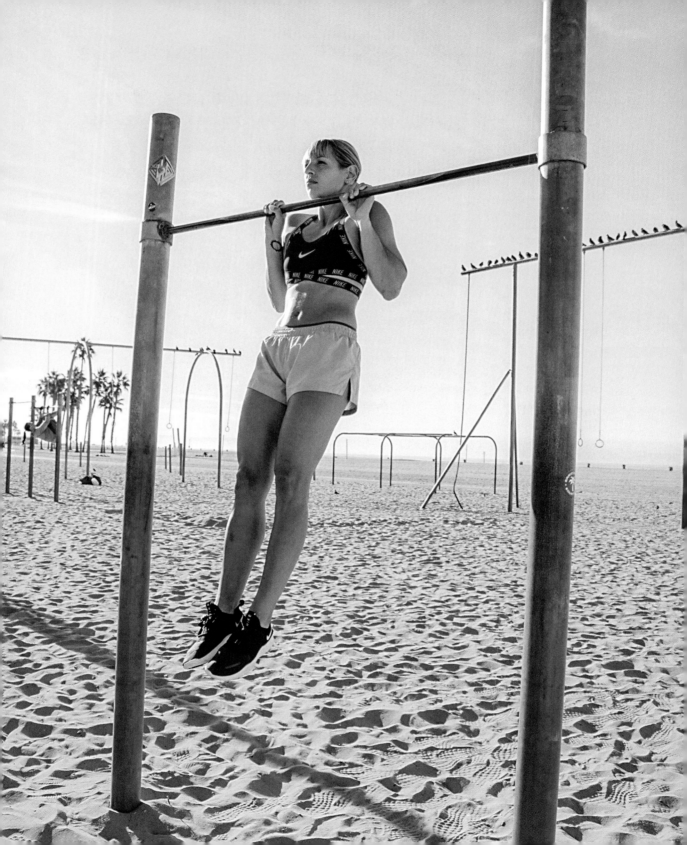

› While you're up there, focus on squeezing your shoulder blades together and engaging your core. Try to hold each flex hang for at least ten seconds.

> *Tip: Flex hangs can also help get you past a plateau if you've been stuck at a certain number of pull-ups for a while. Try adding a few flex hangs for time to the end of your pull-up workout and see just how much stronger you get!*

BODYWEIGHT ROWS

If you know that your biggest current weakness is simply lack of strength, bodyweight rows (also known as reverse push-ups or Australian pull-ups) are a great way to address that.

To do them, you'll need either a low bar about knee height, a dip bar station, or a squat rack with an adjustable bar. You can also do these using gymnastics rings or a TRX. Just be aware that the added instability will make the exercise more difficult.

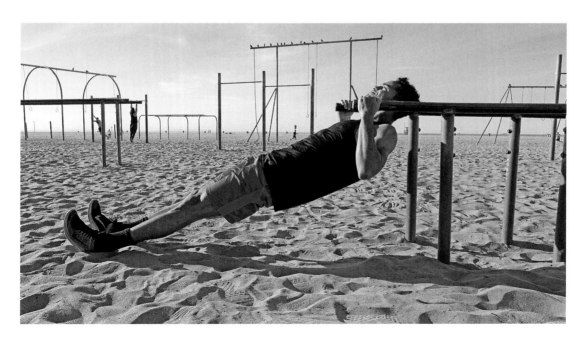

> Lie down under the bar so that your arms are straight and your shoulders are resting just above the floor.
> Straighten your legs and think about bracing your core as well as bringing your shoulders back and down.
> Start with your palms facing toward you in a chin up position, then pull your chest up toward the bar. If this is too hard, go ahead and bend your knees, but try to put as little weight on your legs as you can. You want to rely on your upper-body strength as much as possible to pull your chest toward the bar.

Once you get more comfortable with this movement, you can practice switching grips so that your palms face away from you.

Work up to doing two sets of ten to fifteen bodyweight rows.

JUMPING PULL-UPS

If you can't do a full pull-up yet but flex hangs and bodyweight rows are getting too boring for you, give jumping pull-ups a try.

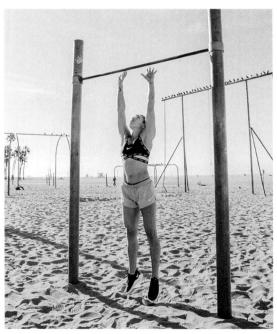 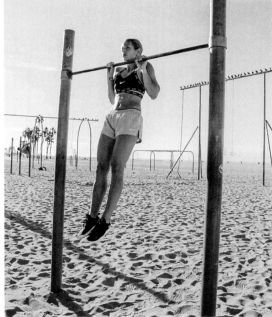

> Stand below a pull-up bar that's too high for you to reach, then lightly jump up and pull yourself up to the bar.

> To make this exercise even more effective, try adding in a slow negative by lowering as slowly as possibly on the way back down.

If you're using a doorway pull-up bar, this is a little trickier but still doable—you'll just need to bend your knees at first in order to get the same benefits.

Work up to doing two sets of eight to ten jumping pull-ups.

BAND-ASSISTED PULL-UPS

Band-assisted pull-ups are a completely optional progression. But they can be a great way to build up strength while continuing to work the other progressions.

Bands can help tremendously in building up the strength needed to do pull-ups because they allow you to perform the full movement while essentially removing some of your own bodyweight to make the exercise easier. Bands can help even the most inexperienced person perform pull-ups, and can be a huge confidence boost. Working with bands can also propel you from doing only one or two pull-ups at a time to doing sets of five, ten, or even more unassisted pull-ups.

The reason that I include this as an optional progression is that sometimes people get stuck using bands forever, and never move on to trying the real thing. This is why if you do choose to include band-assisted pull-ups in your training, I highly recommend also working the other progressions in conjunction with the band work. This way you'll continue to build up strength while also training your mind to actually attempt a full pull-up.

You'll want to start with whatever band allows you to do at least a few pull-ups at a time. When that gets easier (and it will, if you practice), first increase your reps, then graduate to the next-lightest band. If you don't already have bands, you can find them for very reasonable prices online (my favorite are by Rubberbanditz).

To do band-assisted pull-ups, you'll need to first hook the band to the pull-up bar. Do this by looping the band over the pull-up bar, making sure it's secure when you pull it. Grab on to the pull-up bar with both hands and step both feet into the bottom of the band. Pull your shoulders down and back, brace your core, then pull your chest toward the bar before lowering back down.

It's best to practice this with both grips, but you'll probably want to start with a chin up grip since it tends to be easier for most people.

> **Note:** You can keep training with bands even after you're able to do a few unassisted chin-ups or pull-ups. Doing so will help you continue to push past inevitable plateaus in your pull-up training. Once you're able to do ten or more pull-ups with one band, it's time to get a lighter band.

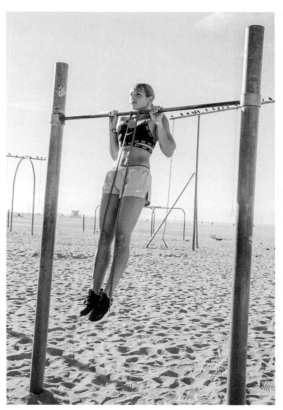
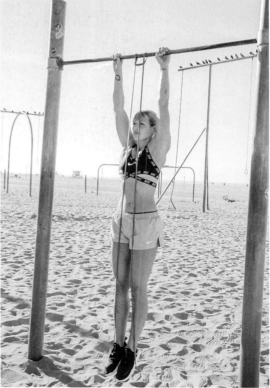

CHIN-UPS

Most people find it easier to start out with their palms facing backward in a chin-up position. This is because chin-ups place more of the burden on your biceps—muscles that most people use on a daily basis and therefore tend to be naturally stronger than the lats and triceps muscles (the muscles used more primarily in pull-ups with your palms facing away from you).

› Hang from a bar with your core tight and your feet hanging slightly in front of you.

› If you have previous shoulder or elbow injuries, you may want to start with your elbows slightly bent, but otherwise begin in a dead hang with your arms completely straight.

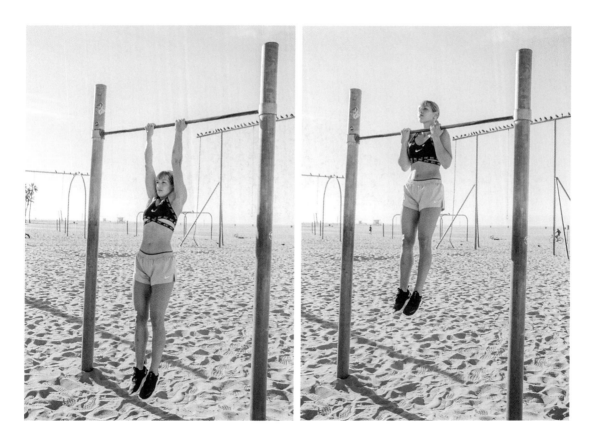

> Pull your shoulders back and down, squeeze everything tight, and pull yourself up to the bar.
> Try to lower down with some control rather than flopping down to avoid unnecessary shoulder injuries.

PULL-UPS

Pull-ups with your hands facing away from you are much harder than chin-ups for most people, so don't feel too discouraged if you can do several chin-ups in a row but can't yet do a single pull-up. Keep practicing your chin-ups, do negatives and jumping pull-ups with your palms facing away from you, and you'll get them with time and patience.

> Grab a bar with a slightly wider grip and face your palms away from you.
> Remember to keep your core tight when doing pull-ups and think about touching your chest to the bar (rather than just trying to get your chin over the bar) before lowering back down.

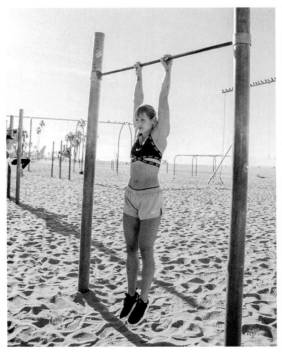 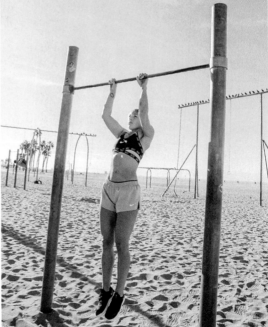

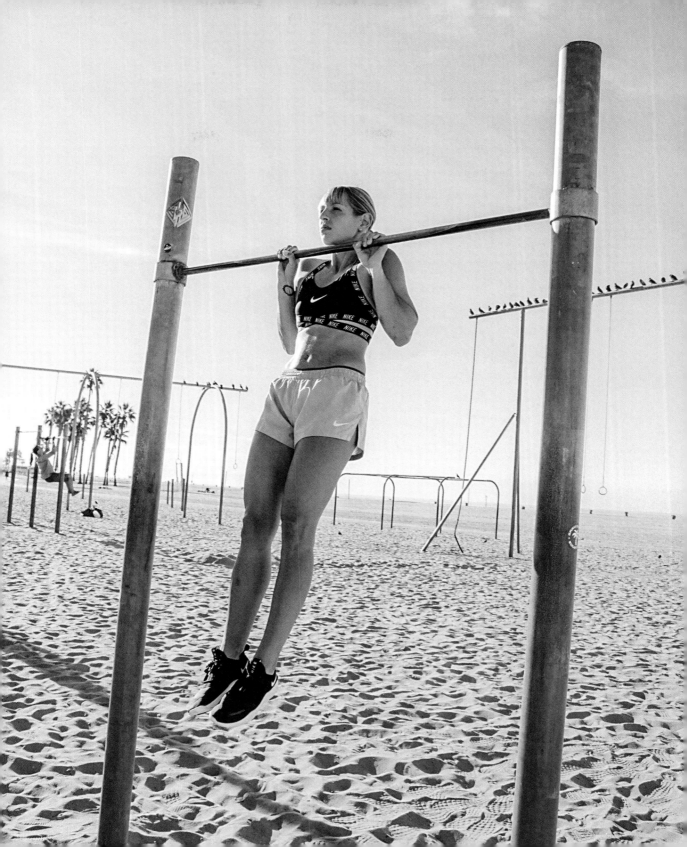

HANGING SCAPULAR SHRUGS

The most-often-skipped part of the pull-up is the initiation from the dead hang that starts with your scapular muscles and is followed by your lats. This is why you may see people do what I call half pull-ups—pull-ups that start with bent arms, and the arms are never fully extended. This makes pull-ups much easier but doesn't count as a full pull-up! Adding hanging scapular shrugs to your workout can help to address this.

To do them, hang from a pull-up bar with your arms completely straight. Relax into this position, then, keeping your arms locked, pull your shoulder blades down while keeping your body tight. Hold briefly, then relax. Aim for control, and don't rush it. The movement will be smaller than you expect.

Aim to do two sets of ten to fifteen before your pull-up training to increase your scapular strength.

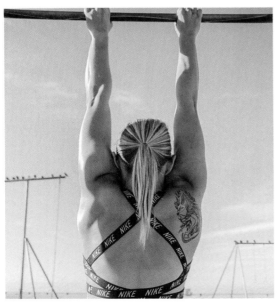
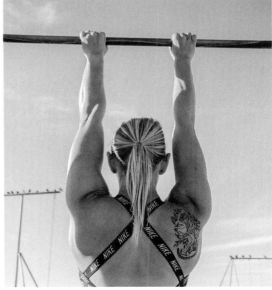

PUSH-UPS: THE MOST UNDERRATED, EFFECTIVE UPPER-BODY EXERCISE EVER

In this age of machines and heavy weights, push-ups tend to be extremely underrated as an exercise. Many traditional weight lifters think they're too good for push-ups, while those who are less strong think they're too difficult to even attempt.

Yet push-ups are one of the best exercises *ever* to work your arms, chest, back, and core muscles. The key to getting the most out of your push-ups is to continuously push yourself to do more difficult versions in order to keep challenging your body to new levels of strength.

Start at whatever level is appropriate for your current strength level, then work up to at least two sets of fifteen before moving on to the next variation.

INCLINE PUSH-UPS

Although most people instinctively drop to their knees when looking for a push-up regression, I'd much rather have you do a full push-up with your hands on an elevated surface. There are two main reasons for this:

› It better mimics a full push-up and allows you to use all the same muscles a regular floor push-up uses.

› It's much easier to gauge your progress when doing incline push-ups, since the lower the surface, the more difficult the push-up becomes.

Here's how to do one:

› Get in front of an elevated surface such as a countertop, table, or bench, then get into a push-up position with your hands on the elevated surface.

› Think about pushing through your shoulders and keeping your core tight and butt squeezed as you lower your chest down until it's almost touching the surface.

› Your elbows can be close to your ribs or slightly flared out, but try not to completely chicken-wing them.

› Push all the way back up, engaging your core and scapular muscles at the top position.

You can continue to increase the difficulty of incline push-ups by doing them on lower and lower surfaces.

Work up to doing two sets of fifteen incline push-ups, continuing to decrease the height as you get stronger.

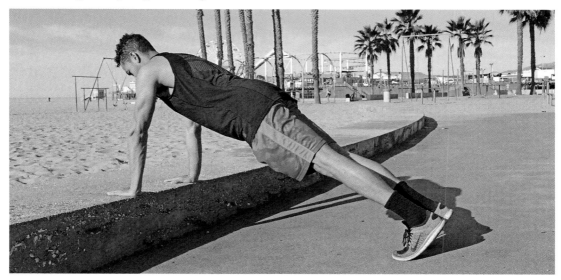

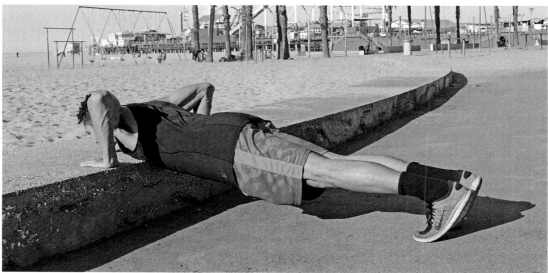

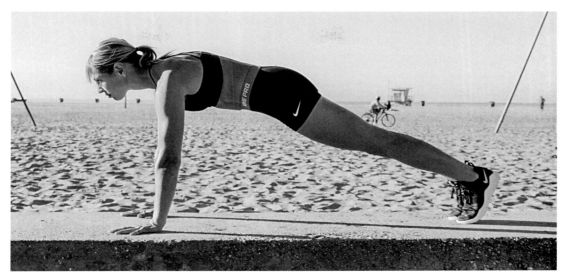

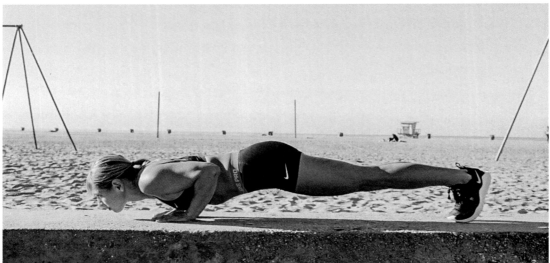

FULL PUSH-UPS

› Get on the floor in a push-up position and think about pushing through your shoulders, squeezing your butt, and keeping your core pulled in as tight as possible.

› Keep your elbows close to your ribs, then lower down so that your chest is no more than a tennis ball's height from the floor before pushing back up.

> If you can't quite get that far yet, don't get discouraged—this is a more difficult push-up than most of us learned growing up, so even those who consider themselves to be pretty strong may have trouble with this one at first.

> When you push back up, remember to push all the way up through your shoulders before beginning the descent again.

Work up to doing two sets of fifteen to twenty full push-ups.

UNEVEN PUSH-UPS

It's a pretty big jump to go from full push-ups to proper one-arm push-ups, so that's where uneven push-ups come in. They start getting your body used to relying mostly on one arm.

As a bonus, they'll help you iron out any imbalances that you may have, such as your right arm being stronger than your left arm (this is very common, so don't worry too much if you discover this is you—uneven push-ups will help balance them out).

To do uneven push-ups, you can use some sort of block (such as a yoga block) or a ball (such as a basketball or medicine ball). The benefit of a ball is that it's easy to move side to side when you're doing these push-ups, and as a bonus makes you look pretty badass.

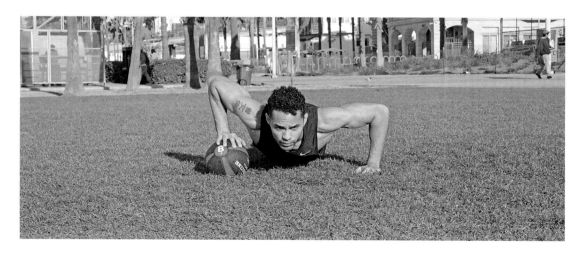

> Get into a push-up position with one hand on the block or ball.
> Lower down so that your chest nearly touches the floor, trying to put as much weight on your non-elevated arm as possible.
> Push back up.

Work up to doing two sets of ten uneven push-ups per side.

ARCHER PUSH-UPS

If your goal is a one arm push-up, archer push-ups are another great way to work on your unilateral arm strength and are a step up from uneven push-ups.

> Get into a push-up position with your arms extended straight out to the sides, perpendicular to your body.
> Squeeze your glutes and leg muscles, brace your core, and don't let your hips sag or pike. Bend one arm and lower your body until your chest nearly touches the floor while keeping your nonworking arm as straight as possible.
> Push back up, then repeat on the opposite side.

Work up to doing two sets of ten archer push-ups per side.

Tip: You can make archer push-ups slightly easier by starting with your hands on an elevated surface similar to an incline push-up.

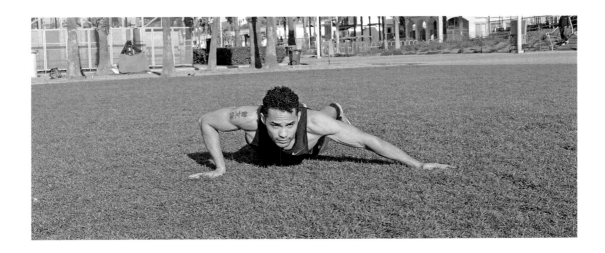

ONE-ARM PUSH-UPS

One-arm push-ups are undoubtedly the most badass push-up of all time, so if you even attempt one, you should be pretty proud of yourself.

› Get into a push-up position, then put one hand behind your back and position yourself over your other hand so that it's straight below your chest.

› You'll probably want to widen your feet a little to make the balancing of this exercise easier.

› Push up through your working shoulder, tighten your core, then lower down as far as possible before pushing back up.

Work up to doing two sets of five one-arm push-ups per side.

OTHER COOL PUSH-UP VARIATIONS TO TRY

There are really an endless number of ways to mix up your push-up training. If you've ever watched advanced calisthenics athletes do push-ups, it's a pretty amazing sight.

Once you master the full push-up, you can not only start working on your one arm push-up progressions but you can also keep trying different push-up styles to mix up your training. Get creative!

Here are some of my favorite push-up variations:

DIAMOND PUSH-UPS
Diamond push-ups emphasize your triceps and just plain look cool.

› Get into a plank position with your hands in a diamond shape in front of you. Your fingers should be touching or almost touching.

› As you lower down, really think about keeping your elbows as close to your body as possible to get the maximum triceps activation out of it.

› Push all the way back up through your shoulders while keeping your core tight.

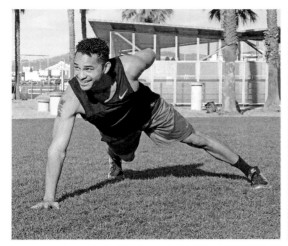
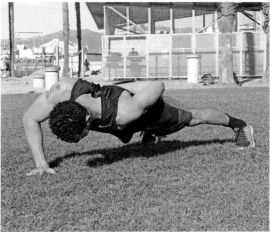
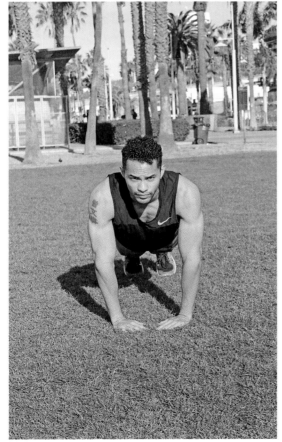
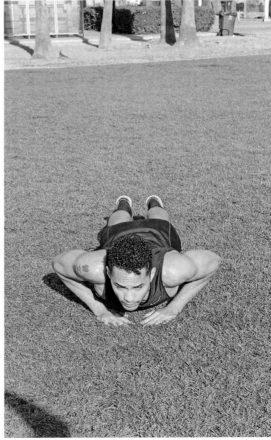

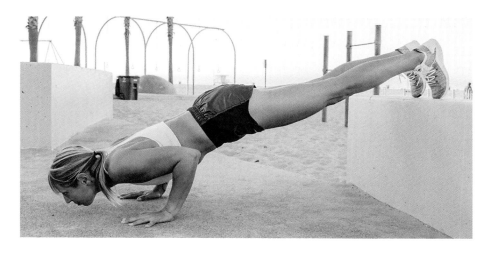

DECLINE PUSH-UPS

› Get into a plank position with your feet on an elevated surface (such as some stairs or a plyo box), then do a push-up.

› The higher the surface, the more challenging this exercise becomes.

REPTILE PUSH-UPS

› Start in a full push-up position, making sure to keep everything tight.

› As you lower your chest to the floor, bring one knee toward your elbow on the same side of the body.

› Push back up into the top of the push-up position and repeat on the opposite side.

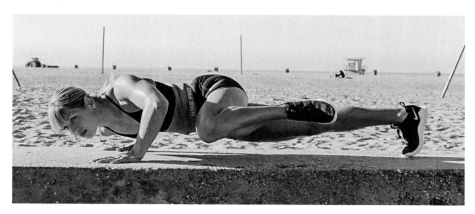

DIVE BOMBER PUSH-UPS

› Start in a downward dog position with your butt piked in the air.
› Bend your elbows and drop your chest to the floor as you push forward to an upward dog position.
› Bend your elbows again, bring your chest back to the floor, then push back up into a downward dog.

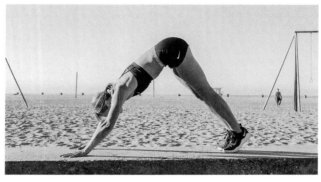

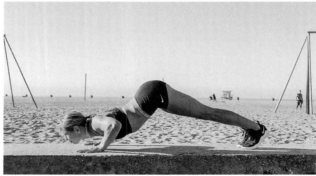

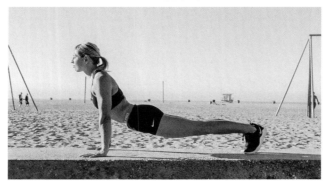

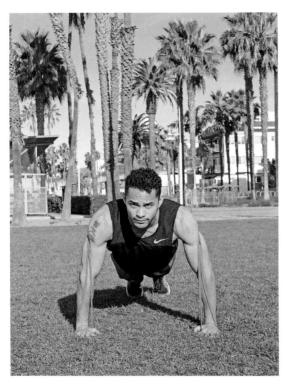 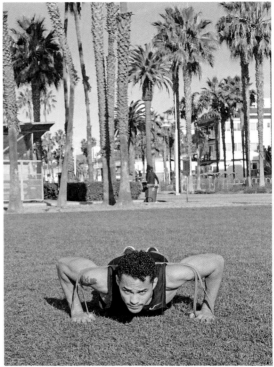

BAND-RESISTED PUSH-UPS
You can add additional resistance to push-ups by adding a band for an extra challenge. This is a great way to push past a plateau if you've been stuck at a certain number of push-ups for a while.

› Start by making an X with the band, place it around your back underneath your arms, and grab one end in each hand.

› Get into a push-up position with your shoulders directly over your hands and your arms close to your sides.

› Lower your chest down toward the floor, focusing on keeping your body straight and your core tight as you push back up.

PLYOMETRIC PUSH-UPS
See the section on plyometric push-ups beginning on page 153.

DIPS FOR TRICEPS OF STEEL

Triceps dips are one of the best and most underutilized exercises for building a strong upper body and helping you prepare for even more advanced calisthenics exercises like muscle-ups and handstand push-ups.

Not only will dips build up your triceps strength like no other exercise can, they'll also work the front of your shoulders (anterior deltoids), your chest (pectorals), and your rhomboids, as well as your abdominal muscles to build core strength.

Plus, they'll get you more functionally strong than any machine-assisted triceps exercise *ever* will. These should be a staple part of your training regimen, no matter your current fitness level.

GETTING STARTED WITH TRICEPS DIPS

Although a lot of gymgoers are familiar with the modified bench dip, most people don't actually know the best way to scale up the exercise and build up to the full-range-of-motion triceps dip. The progressions over the next few pages will help you safely build up the strength you need to get there.

Start with whichever progression is appropriate for your current strength level. For all the following dip progressions, you'll want to be able to do ten to fifteen clean reps before you move on to the next progression (although that doesn't mean you can't try the harder versions for fun as you go along—just be smart and don't do anything that hurts!).

CORRECT PARALLEL BAR WIDTH (AND HOW TO AVOID SHOULDER INJURIES)

You may have heard that triceps dips put you at risk for a shoulder or rotator cuff injury and should be avoided. But the main reason that people end up injuring themselves when doing triceps dips is not that the exercise itself is risky but that they're using incorrect form and bars that are too wide for their stature.

In fact, although parallel bars at outdoor fitness parks and gyms are great pieces of equipment, they're almost always too wide for the average person doing triceps dips. If you've ever felt awkward or that your shoulders are hurting when trying to do triceps dips on parallel bars, this is most likely why.

The correct width for triceps dips should be approximately the length of your forearm from elbow to fingertips, and no wider. Just for reference, most parallel bars are at least 25 percent too wide for most people!

This is why having adjustable bars or using gymnastics rings can be a safer option when working the triceps dip.

BENT-KNEE BENCH DIPS

If you're just starting out with dips, bench knee dips are a great way to begin to build up your triceps strength and are the version of dips that most people are more familiar with.

› Get in front of a bench or sturdy elevated surface and position your hands palms down on the bench behind you.
› Your legs should be bent in front of you and your feet on the ground. Pull your shoulders back and keep your chest high, then lower down so that your elbows are at a 90-degree angle.
› Push back up and repeat.

Work up to doing two sets of twenty-five bench knee dips.

STRAIGHT-LEG BENCH DIPS

Once you're fairly comfortable with bench knee dips, it's time to move on to straight leg bench dips.

› You'll want to get in a similar position as with the bench knee dips but with your legs extended straight on the ground.
› Engage your core, pull your shoulders back, and lower down so that your

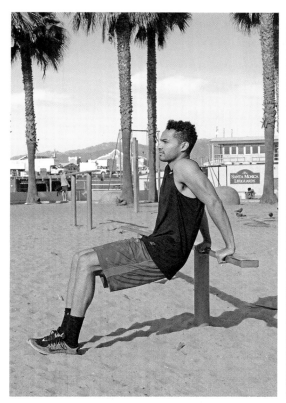
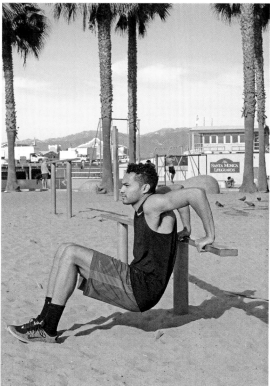
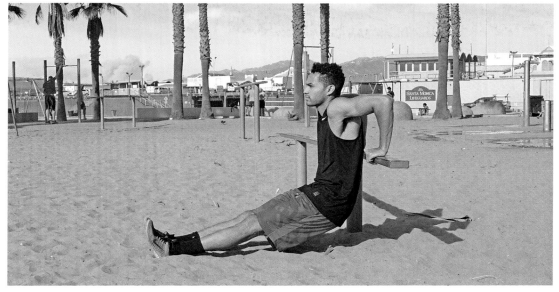

elbows are parallel with the floor.

Work up to doing two to three sets of twenty-five straight-leg bench dips.

ASSISTED TRICEPS DIPS

The next step in the dip progression is to do dips using assistance from one leg. This gets significantly harder, so don't worry if it's difficult for you at first—you'll build up strength quickly with practice! You'll need a set of parallel bars or an equivalent to do these.

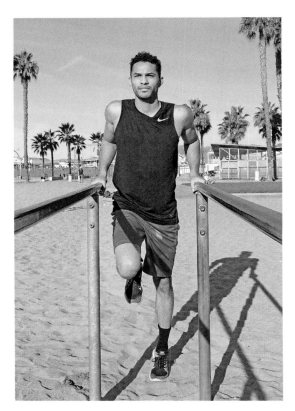

You can also do these either in front of a bench with one leg on a bench or chair in front of you, or you can put your leg up on a set of p-bars with the other leg lightly resting on the ground.

› If you're using a bench, try to get to parallel, making sure to switch legs every so often.

› If you're using p-bars, try to get to below a 90-degree angle and make sure to lean forward slightly as you lower down to keep your shoulders healthy and happy.

Work up to doing two sets of fifteen one-elevated-leg bench dips.

BAND-ASSISTED TRICEPS DIPS

If you're feeling stuck in the one-leg-elevated version of triceps dips, using a band for support may help you push past that plateau. The lighter the band, the more of your own bodyweight you'll be using (and the harder the exercise will feel).

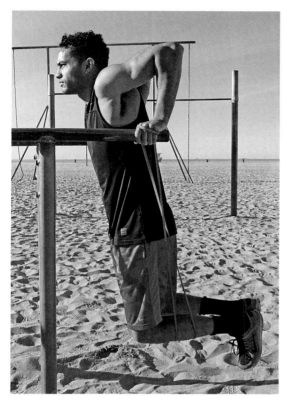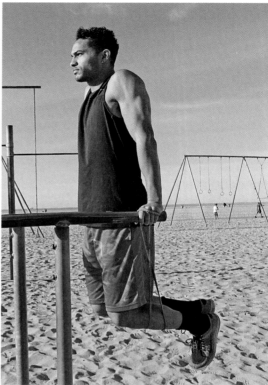

> Grasp each end of the band around the bar and rest your knees on top of it.

> Keep your chest up and shoulders back as you lower yourself down as far as you can.

> Push yourself back up to starting position.

FULL RANGE OF MOTION TRICEPS DIPS

> For full triceps dips, get in between a dip bar or a set of p-bars. Grip the bars at your side.

> Push up through your shoulders, engage your core, and lean forward slightly while keeping your chest upright.

> As you lower down, you can either cross your legs or straighten them and bring them at an angle in front of you to keep them off the ground.

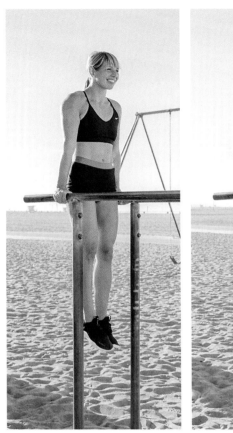
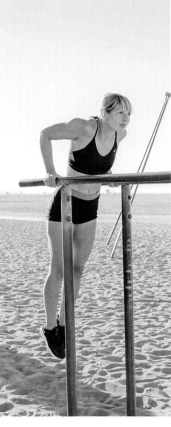
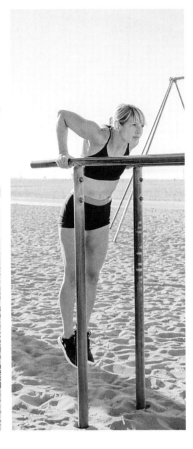

There is some contention among trainers about which leg position is preferable, but the straight-leg version undoubtedly leads to fewer shoulder injuries, so if you have the space, try it that way.

On full range of motion dips, you want to try to get to at least a 90-degree angle with your elbows. But don't stop there—your ultimate goal is actually to be able to go all the way down so that the bars are basically at your armpits before pushing back up.

DIP BAR SUBSTITUTES

Don't have access to parallel bars or a dip bar station? There are still plenty of ways to work your triceps dips—you just have to get a little creative. Here are several equipment substitutions to try for triceps dips, L-sits, and other traditional parallel bar exercises:

› Place two stools or tall chairs together. Your hands will be on the chair seats as you perform the dips.

› If you have a spot in your kitchen where two counters come together perpendicularly you can use that corner spot as a makeshift dip station. For triceps dips, you'll actually be facing the countertops and performing dips with your arms at a slight angle.

› Look around you—there are many more dip bar equivalents outside than you might realize. Playgrounds and even bike racks are often great substitutes.

› Get some gymnastics rings and hang them from a sturdy tree, a swing set, or even a basketball hoop and work your dips. Just be aware that rings will make any exercise more difficult because of the added instability.

OTHER COOL DIP VARIATIONS TO TRY

Once you've mastered the full triceps dip, the possibilities are endless. Although you'll first want to put your energy into training for multiple reps and make sure you've got your form down, here are some other fun dip variations you can try:

BAND-RESISTED TRICEPS DIPS
While most people use workout bands to make exercises like pull-ups and triceps dips easier, you can also use bands to add more resistance to exercises like triceps dips.

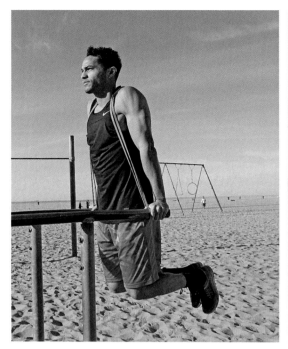 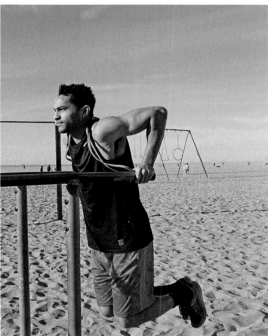

> › Place the middle of the band around the back of your neck and grasp each end in a hand to add resistance to your dips as you ascend.
> › Straighten your arms and raise your legs off the ground. Keep your chest up and shoulders back as you lower yourself down as far as you can.
> › Finally, press yourself back up to the starting position.

STRAIGHT BAR DIPS
> › Position both hands in front of your body on a single straight bar.
> › Lower yourself down as you lean over the bar and reach your legs out in front to keep your balance.

Straight bar dips require more shoulder, bicep, and abdominal strength as well as a greater sense of balance—so don't be discouraged if they feel extra tough at first.

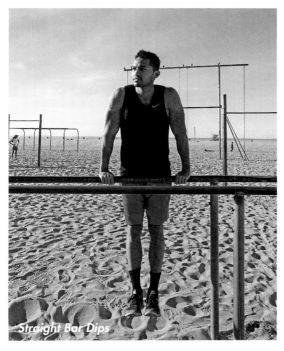

Straight Bar Dips

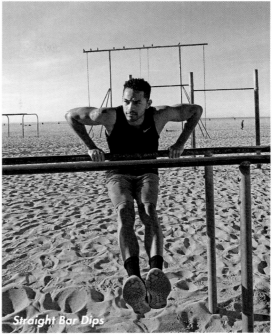

Straight Bar Dips

KOREAN DIPS

›   Position both hands behind your body on a single straight bar.

›   Engage your abs and dip down so that your elbows reach at least 90 degrees, then push back up.

The Korean dip is an extremely challenging variation of the dip—you should be fairly comfortable with regular straight bar dips and be able to do at least fifteen regular triceps dips before you even give it a try.

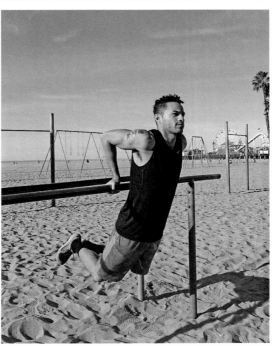

RING DIPS
Adding rings to your triceps dips adds a whole other level of difficulty, since not only do you have to still do a dip but you also have to constantly stabilize yourself while in that position.

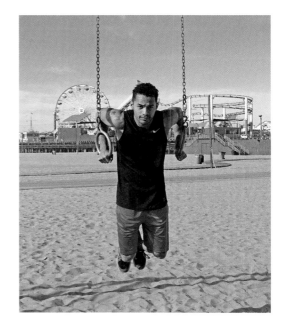

› You'll first need to boost yourself up on the rings, holding them at your sides with your palms facing toward your body and your thumbs facing slightly outward.

› Slowly lower down as you turn your thumbs facing forward, holding your legs in front of you in a hollow position (or bent if space doesn't allow for straight legs) with your chest upright.

› You want to aim for a 90-degree angle or below, but if you can only get a few inches down at first, that's okay—just stick with it and you *will* get stronger!

GET UPSIDE DOWN WITH HANDSTANDS

If you've been following me on my blog or on social media at all for the past few years, you probably know I'm very passionate about handstands.

But unless you were there at the beginning (and some of you were), you might not understand just how far I've come in my handstand journey. Although bystanders will often stop and ask whether I'm a gymnast during my workout these days, nothing could be further from the truth. In fact, before I started working on my handstands around four years ago, I had absolutely no experience in hand balancing, gymnastics, or anything even remotely related.

I decided to learn to handstand because it seemed like one of the most difficult things I could do. I wanted to prove to myself that with hard work and consistency, I could do something that felt nearly impossible when first starting out.

Along the way, I've absolutely fallen in love with handstands and everything related to them. I'm constantly working to improve my skills and am always seeking out more experienced teachers to help my personal handstand journey as well as to help my own clients and readers to discover a love of handstands.

Because of all this, handstands have a very special place in my heart, and I love to encourage anyone with even the slightest bit of interest to start working on them. If you've never done a handstand in your life, a freestanding handstand may sound far-fetched to you right now. But with the right progressions, hard work, and patience, you, too, can do a handstand if you put your mind to it.

WHY I BELIEVE EVERYONE SHOULD LEARN TO HANDSTAND

Yes, they're a cool party trick and will definitely impress your friends. But handstands have a lot of other benefits as well:

› THEY BUILD CORE AND UPPER BODY STRENGTH. Handstands work more than a dozen muscles in your body, including muscles in your back, chest, arms, wrists, core, and even glutes. Training them regularly will really help to strengthen these muscles.

› THEY HELP WITH BONE HEALTH, CIRCULATION, AND BREATHING. When you're upside down in a handstand, your normal blood flow inverts, increasing circulation to your upper body while relieving pressure on your feet and legs. Handstands also benefit your spine, increase bone health in your wrists, arms, and shoulders, and stretch your diaphragm, your main breathing muscle, which in turn increases blood flow to your lungs.

› THEY CAN BOOST YOUR MOOD AND REGULATE YOUR METABOLISM. Being upside down not only makes you stronger but it can actually boost your mood, since the extra blood flow to your brain can energize and calm you when you're feeling down or stressed out. Handstands can even reduce production of the stress hormone cortisol, helping to relieve minor depression and anxiety. Plus, since handstands stimulate the thyroid and pituitary glands, they can actually help regulate your metabolic rate—meaning daily handstand practice could help you reach or maintain a healthy weight.

AVOIDING THE "BANANA HANDSTAND" AGAINST THE WALL

If you've ever tried a handstand against the wall before, you've more than likely placed your hands on the floor, then kicked your feet up so that your back is against the wall.

Although this may feel like the easiest way to get into a handstand, I actually want you to avoid this as much as possible when you're new to practicing handstands. The reason for this is that this way of practicing will more likely than not teach your body to hold what's known in the hand balancing world as the "banana handstand"—a handstand where your body is arched like a banana, rather than stacked and straight like a ruler.

Not only does this result in an extremely inefficient handstand (meaning it takes more strength to hold) but it also makes it much harder to actually balance once you're at the point where you're working on freestanding handstands.

Learning to avoid the banana handstand early on will make your handstand training much easier down the road.

GETTING STARTED WITH HANDSTANDS

The following progressions will help you build up to a freestanding handstand, no matter where you're starting from. Be patient, and practice often—consistency is key with handstands!

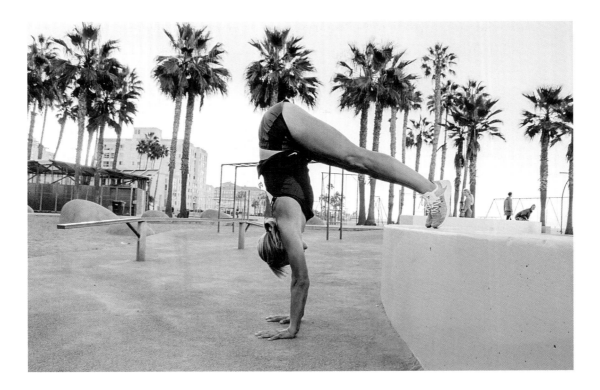

HALF-HANDSTAND HOLD

If you're brand-new to handstands, even the idea of going fully vertical may be intimidating at first. These half-handstand holds will help you build strength and endurance and get your body used to being partially inverted.

> Find a bench, a couple of steps, or something a little lower than waist high, then place your feet on the elevated surface and your hands down on the ground.

> Walk your hands back until your hips are stacked directly over your shoulders, or as far as you can go.

> Engage your core, push up through your shoulders, and hold this position. Work up to three sets of thirty-second holds.

CHEST-TO-WALL HANDSTAND

The first step in being able to hold a freestanding handstand is to spend a lot of

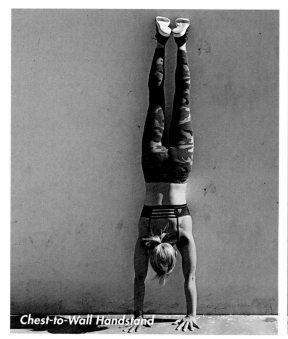

Chest-to-Wall Handstand

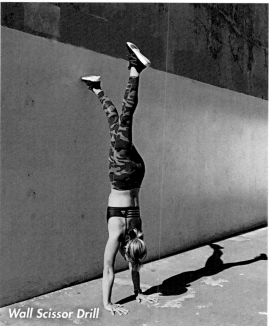

Wall Scissor Drill

time on the wall. It may not seem very cool or overly impressive, but working your wall handstand is absolutely essential to building up strength and endurance upside down, as well as helping you to establish a solid handstand line.

Instead of kicking up against the wall like most people do, walk your feet up the wall so that your chest touches the wall. This makes it much easier to establish a straight handstand line at the very beginning and will help you avoid the bad habit of an arched "banana handstand" later on.

› Place your hands in front of the wall, then slowly walk your feet up the wall until you reach vertical. Your goal is to get your hands a few inches away from the wall. If you can't quite get that close to the wall yet, don't worry—part of this initial training is learning to understand the feeling of being upside down. It will get better with time and practice.

› Once you reach the right position, tighten your core, pull your ribs in, and push up as much as possible through your shoulders. You should feel like you're pushing the floor away from you.

> Next, point your toes, engage your glutes and quads, and hold! Try to do at least three sets of holds and time yourself to track your improvement.

Work up to holding a wall handstand for three sets of forty-five to sixty seconds. When you start feeling more comfortable upside down, try to practice removing your feet from the wall for as long as possible before cartwheeling or walking back down.

WALL SCISSOR DRILL

Once you feel more comfortable being upside down and can hold your wall handstand for at least forty-five seconds, you can start working on the balance portion of the handstand.

Rather than going straight to working on your freestanding handstand, you can still use the wall as a tool to help you get the feeling of balance in your fingertips and understand the proper handstand line you should be aiming for when freestanding. This wall scissor drill is one of my favorites for starting to understand the correct stacking position in a handstand.

Start by walking up the wall into a handstand. Make sure everything is tight and really push up through your shoulders.

Next, walk your hands away from the wall so that they're about a foot or so away. Your hips should still be over your hands.

Slowly remove one foot from the wall and balance it overhead so that your shoulders and hips remain in a straight line. It's okay if your leg goes slightly past your hips; just really make sure to focus on your hips being directly over your shoulders.

With as much control as possible, slowly remove the other foot from the wall and try to balance through your fingers and hold your handstand briefly. If you fall backward, just put your feet back on the wall. If you fall forward, just cartwheel out. Part of learning handstands is learning that falling is okay!

Very slowly split your legs back and forth, working to feel the balance in your fingertips and the alignment in your shoulders and hips.

Try to film yourself during this exercise regularly to gauge your progress. And don't rush it. Gaining balance takes time!

FREESTANDING HANDSTAND

As soon as you can hold yourself up in a wall handstand for forty-five seconds or more, you can start practicing your freestanding handstands. The longer you can hold it against the wall, the easier working on your freestanding handstand will be.

Keep in mind that freestanding handstands without a wall are *significantly* harder than wall handstands.

Not only do they require enough strength and endurance to hold yourself upside down, they also mean you need to have good proprioception (an understanding of where your body is in space), as well as an awareness of how to balance in a vertical position. Although some people can build up to a freestanding handstand within a few months of practicing, others can expect it to take a year or more before everything begins to click. Be patient with yourself, and try to enjoy the process.

You can experiment with either kicking into a handstand or jumping up into a handstand. Most people will find kick-ups easier since jumping up with two legs takes a lot of upper back and shoulder flexibility.

When kicking up, go slowly! This takes a lot of experimenting. If you don't kick hard enough, you won't make it to vertical, and if you kick too hard, you'll fall or cartwheel over. Again, be patient with the process. It takes time and practice.

Just like with the wall scissor drill, try to feel the balance in your fingertips and focus on keeping your shoulders and hips stacked over your hands and pulling your ribs in to avoid arching your back.

When you do feel ready to start training your handstands away from the wall, don't stop your wall training altogether. Even the best hand balancers often still work on the wall to gain even more strength and endurance and work on perfecting their handstand line.

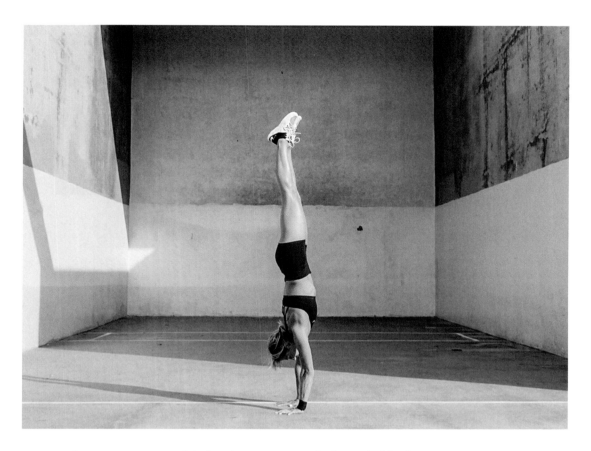

Once you get to this level, try to spend about half of your time practicing your handstand on the wall and half of your time working on kicking up into a freestanding handstand. Only when you get really consistent holding your freestanding handstand for a minute or more should you start spending most or all of your time off of the wall.

Learning to handstand without a wall can be incredibly frustrating and humbling, but don't get discouraged! With time and consistent practice, you *will* be able to hold a freestanding handstand. Determination, focus on form, and constantly adjusting for mistakes will get you there.

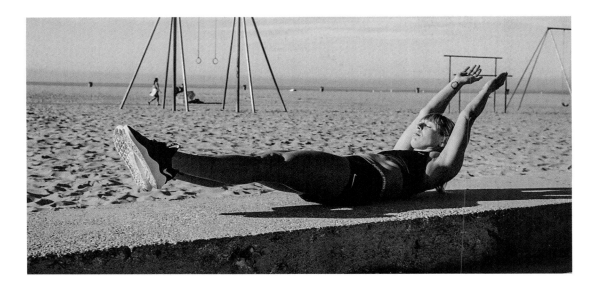

OTHER HELPFUL HANDSTAND DRILLS

The following drills will help you build strength and endurance as well as begin the process of finding balance in a handstand.

HOLLOW-BODY HOLDS

The hollow-body shape is the same shape you ultimately want to hold in a handstand. Adding these to your handstand training will help you engage the same muscles as you would while upside down, as well as help you build a super-strong core.

To do them, lie down on your back and contract your abs, pulling your belly button toward the floor. Your arms and legs should be held straight out from your body with your hands and toes pointing away from you.

Slowly raise your shoulders and legs from the ground as you keep your lower back in contact with the floor. The goal is to find the lowest position that you can hold your arms and legs in without breaking lower back contact.

If this is too tough at first, you can modify it by reaching your hands toward your feet, and make it even easier by tucking your knees toward your chest.

Work up to doing three sets of forty-five-second holds.

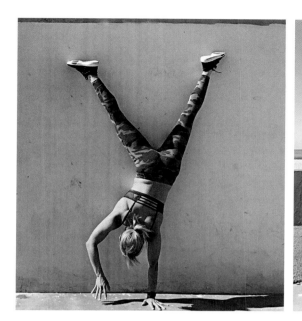 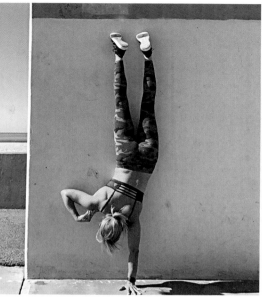

WALL WALKS

Wall walks are a great exercise to help build up your strength and endurance in a handstand and get you used to the feeling of being upside down. To do them, walk your feet up the wall so that your chest is close to the wall, and then pick one hand up as you walk in one direction.

Slightly straddle your legs, tighten your core, and push up through your shoulders. Lean to one side as you step your hand in that same direction and allow your hips and feet to follow. Make sure to work both directions.

Work up to two sets of sixty seconds of wall walks.

SHOULDER TOUCHES

This is another great strengthener and really helps you focus on that necessary shoulder push in a handstand. Plus, it can help prepare you for a one-arm handstand way down the line.

Once you're in a handstand against the wall, lean slightly to one side as you slowly pick one hand up. You can start by just moving your fingertips to understand the movement, then eventually work up to touching your shoulder on the same side. Handstand shoulder touches are great to do for time or reps in addition to your wall holds.

Work up to doing two sets of thirty to forty shoulder touches.

BEYOND THE HANDSTAND: HANDSTAND PUSH-UPS

Even if you start to enjoy—and get good at—handstands, handstand push-ups are still incredibly intimidating for most people. In fact, the majority of people think handstand push-ups are near impossible—that they're only for gymnast types with insanely broad shoulders and strong and compact bodies.

But just like anything else, if you work the right progressions and are consistent with your training, you *can* do handstand push-ups. Yes, you might have a harder time if you have longer arms (my nickname for years was "Spaghetti Arms," so I can relate), or if your back and shoulder muscles aren't already fairly strong.

Yes, it will take time to build up the strength and coordination to do them. But even just working the regressions will do wonders to strengthen your upper body and core muscles. With time and patience, you'll be able to do the full thing.

THE AWESOME BENEFITS OF HANDSTAND PUSH-UPS

Not only do they look really impressive but handstand push-ups (and all the regressions) also provide a number of awesome benefits:

- They target your bent-arm strength, a perfect complement to the straight-arm strength of handstands
- They build incredible shoulder and upper-body strength
- They also work your core, glutes, and even quadriceps muscles
- They make you feel like a (really strong) kid!

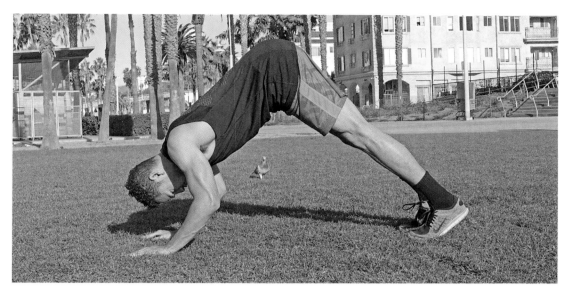

HANDSTAND PUSH-UP PROGRESSIONS

If you follow the progression of exercises on the next few pages, you'll build the technique, strength, and confidence necessary to be able to do handstand push-ups.

Start wherever is the most appropriate for your current fitness level. If you're not sure where you're at, begin at the first progression and go from there. Then make sure to include these exercises in your workout routine two to three times a week for the fastest possible results.

BENT-ARM BEAR

If you're starting from the very beginning and need to build up strength, holding the bent-arm bear position is the best place to start.

› Start in an inverted pike position with your hands under your shoulders and your knees under your hips.

› Push your butt up high as you bend through your arms while keeping your legs as straight as possible.

› Focus on keeping your elbows in and loading the front of your body as much as possible as you hold for time.

Work up to holding this position for three sets of twenty-second holds.

PIKE PUSH-UPS

Once you can hold the bent-arm bear position for time, the next step is to work your pike push-ups (also called inverted presses).

> Get in an inverted pike position with your hands under your shoulders and knees under your hips.

> Push your butt up as high as you can, and step your feet slightly closer to your hands.

> Lean forward and load your weight over your hands as you rotate your elbow pits forward.

> Squeeze your elbows together as you bend your arms, aiming to touch your head on the floor in front of you so that it forms a triangle with your hands.

> Keep your core tight as you push back up to the starting position.

If you're struggling to get back up from the floor, you can start by placing a mat or yoga block in front of your hands to lessen the distance. You can also work the negative portion of the pike push-up to help build up strength.

Work up to doing three sets of six to eight reps.

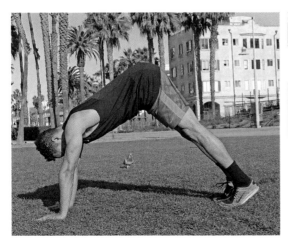
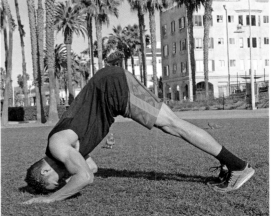

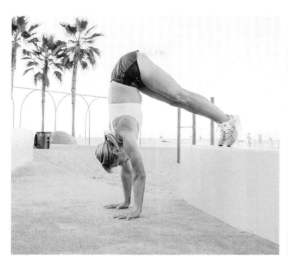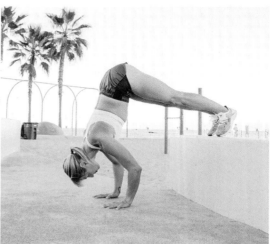

FEET-ELEVATED PIKE PUSH-UPS

When you feel pretty comfortable doing pike push-ups on the floor, it's time to up the challenge by elevating your feet.

› Find a sturdy surface that's about waist high or slightly lower.

› Set your feet on the surface and place your hands on the floor, thinking about keeping a 90-degree position.

› Bend your arms and lower your forehead down to the imaginary triangle in front of your hands.

› Focus on keeping your core tight and elbows squeezed together as you lower down, then raise back up.

Work up to three sets of six to eight reps.

WALL HANDSTAND PUSH-UPS

Once you're feeling pretty good about your feet-elevated pike push-ups, it's time to get to the fun stuff: handstand push-ups against a wall.

› Get into a handstand position with your chest facing the wall, then walk your hands forward a couple of feet.

› Squeeze your core, glutes, and thighs as much as possible, and lower your forehead down to the imaginary triangle in front of your hands, keeping your elbows close to your ribs as you do so.

› You'll probably want to start by putting a mat or yoga block in front of your hands so that you have less of a chance of crashing onto the hard floor.

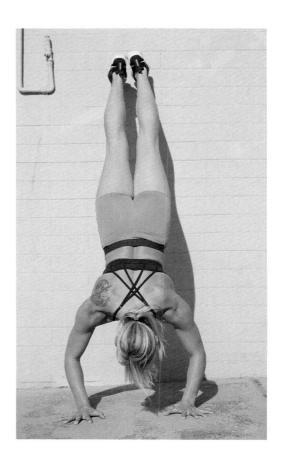

You can also work the negative portion of the wall handstand push-up to build up strength. If you do this, make sure to go as slowly as possible to get the most out of the movement.

Work up to three sets of five or more reps.

FREESTANDING HANDSTAND PUSH-UPS

Your ultimate goal for handstand push-ups? To be able to do them without a wall. Yes, this may seem fairly unattainable for the average person right now, but if you keep working your handstands and handstand push-ups variation, you'll get there eventually.

You should be able to hold a freestanding handstand for at least ten seconds before attempting freestanding handstand push-ups.

› Get into a handstand, then lower your forehead down to the imaginary triangle in front of your hands.

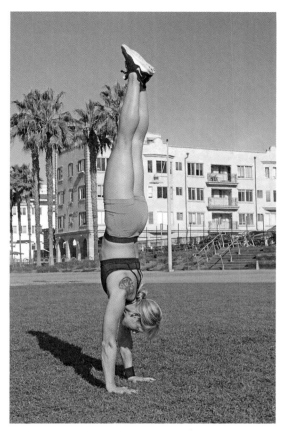 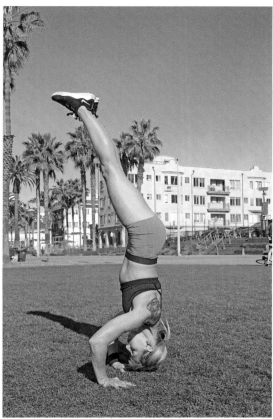

› Your feet should remain slightly piked behind you and your core should be tight.

› Push back up.

Don't be surprised if your back bends a little more on this one at first to compensate for the lack of wall balance—your form will improve with time and practice.

Remember: skills like handstand push-ups take years for most people to perfect, so don't get discouraged if you can't do a perfect one in the first few weeks or even months. Keep working on them and slowly but surely you'll build up strength and confidence.

WRIST STRETCHES AND STRENGTHENERS

When you first start doing handstands, you may notice that your wrists start to ache and get stiff and sore. This is normal, and it just means that you're using your wrists a lot more than usual. For some people, this never ends up being too much of a problem, since practicing handstands regularly will naturally strengthen your wrists. But most people need a little extra strengthening and stretching in order to reduce any wrist pain that comes with doing a lot of handstands and other upper-body exercises.

These wrist exercises may seem boring at first, but trust me, they'll work wonders to help keep your wrists strong, flexible, and injury-free. Make it a habit to do one to two sets before practicing handstands or other wrist-centric exercises to strengthen and loosen up your wrists. During each of these exercises, make sure to move gently and never push to the point where you feel pain. As your fingers and wrists get stronger, you'll notice that your handstands start improving as well.

HANDS FACING AWAY FROM YOU (PALMS DOWN)
› Kneel on the ground with your hands on the ground, palms down and fingers facing away from you.
› Lightly rock back and forth so that you feel a stretch in the inside of your wrists, as well as a loosening up of the front of your wrists.
› Do ten reps.

HANDS FACING TOWARD YOU (PALMS UP)
› Rock back and forth so that you feel a light stretch on the outside of your wrists.
› Do ten reps.

HANDS FACING TOWARD YOU (PALMS DOWN)
› Rock back and forth so that you feel a light stretch on the inside of your wrists.
› Do ten reps.

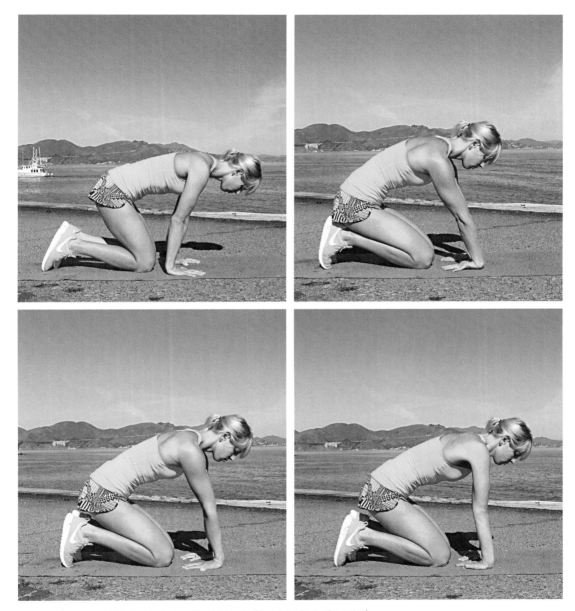

FINGERS FACING SIDEWAYS (PALMS DOWN)

› Place your palms down with your fingers facing in toward one another.

› Slowly rock one direction, then circle back to the starting position.

› Do five circles to one side, then switch directions.

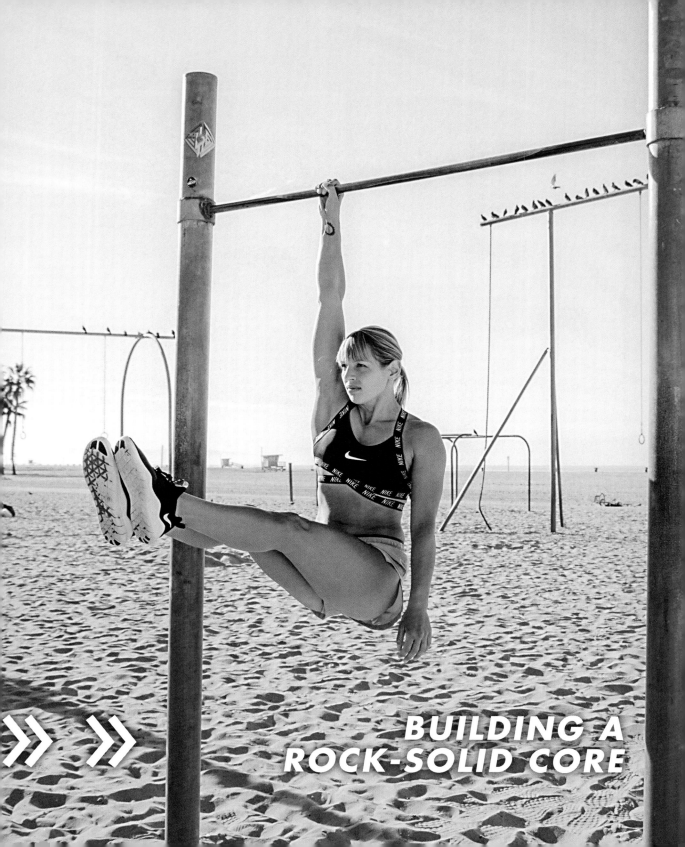

BUILDING A
ROCK-SOLID CORE

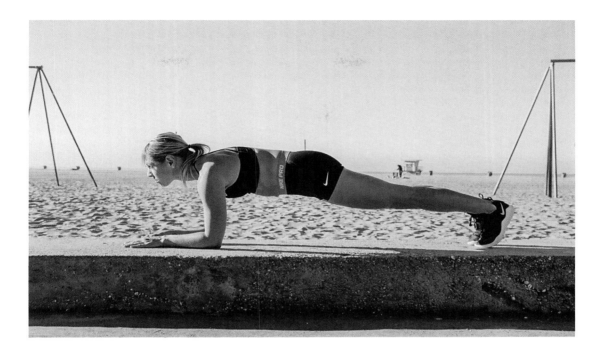

FOREARM PLANK

Forearm planks are the first progression to building a strong core, and put more of an emphasis on your abs than some of the later plank progressions do. For that reason, you can continue to do forearm planks even after progressing to the harder versions if you want—although you'll have to hold them for longer periods of time or add in some instability to continue making progress.

> Get in a plank position with your shoulders directly over your hands and your forearms on the floor.
> Your hands can be facing slightly forward or angled into more of a triangle.
> Lift your hips so that your back is slightly rounded, squeeze your core, and push through your shoulders.
> Continue to engage your core, glutes, and leg muscles, and keep a neutral chin as you hold the position for time.

Work toward three rounds of forty-five-second holds.

HIGH PLANK

› Get in a plank position with your hands on the floor, directly under your shoulders.

› Push away from the floor as you squeeze your abs, glutes, and leg muscles and hold the position.

› Don't let your hips sag or pike up!

Work toward three rounds of forty-five-second holds.

ONE-ARM PLANK

› Get in a full plank position, making sure to pull your core in and keep everything tight.

› Step your feet out slightly so that they're in a narrow straddle stance.

› Think about keeping your hips in one place as you raise one arm and slowly lift it off the ground, resting it behind your back.

› Push up as much as possible through your working arm.

Work toward three rounds of twenty-five-second holds per arm.

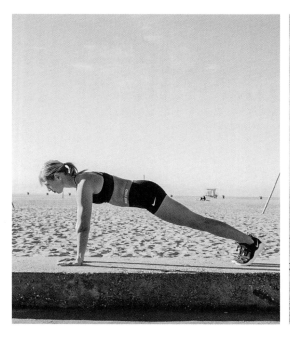 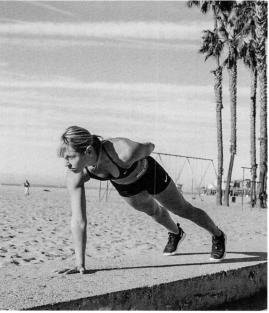

OTHER PLANK VARIATIONS

Although standard planks should always have a place in your workouts, there's no question that holding planks for longer and longer periods of time can get a little boring. Here are some interesting ways to add variety to your planks:

ELEVATED KNEE TOUCHES

› Start in a plank position with your feet on a box or elevated surface with your hands on the floor in front of you.

› Tighten your core and push through your shoulders, then bring one knee toward your elbow on the same side.

› Return your leg to the starting position and repeat on the other side.

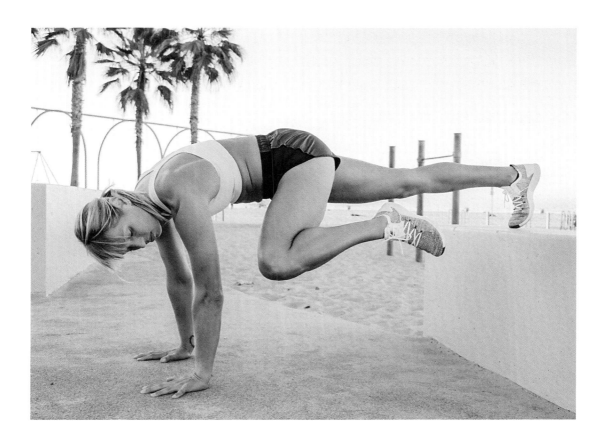

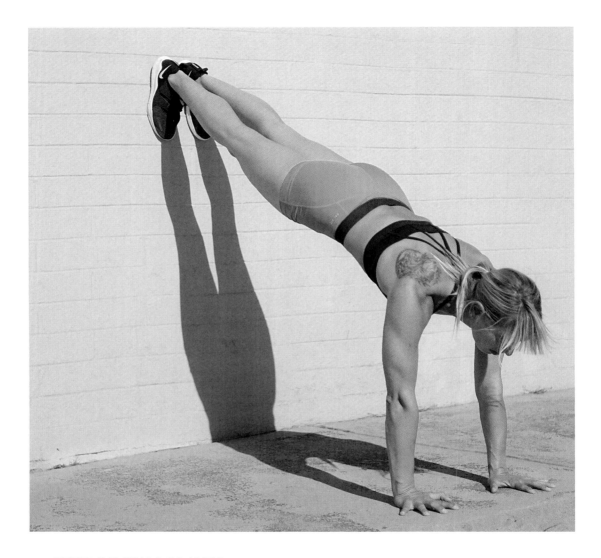

FEET-ON-WALL PLANKS

› Get in front of a wall; place your hands on the floor and your feet on the
  wall.

› Walk your hands out until your shoulders are directly over your hands in
  a plank position.

› Push up through your shoulders and hold for time.

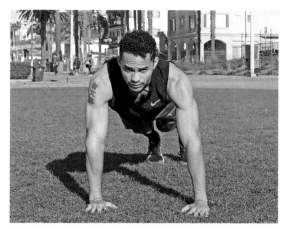 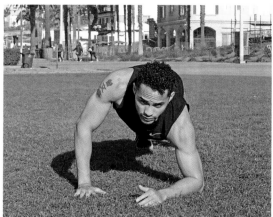

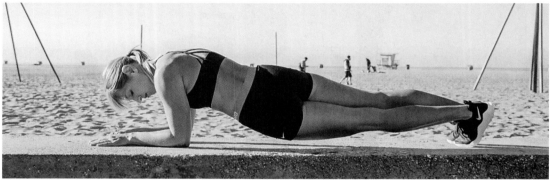

PLANK GET-UPS

› Get into a plank position with your shoulders directly over your hands.

› Lower down to your elbow on one side, then follow with the other side.

› Straighten one arm and then the other until you're back in the starting plank position.

› Switch starting arms and repeat.

PLANK HIP DIPS

› Get into a forearm plank, then swivel your torso to one side, bringing your hip down until it touches the floor.

› Return to the top plank position, then swivel your torso to the opposite side.

› Make sure to keep your core tight the entire time. Each side counts as one rep.

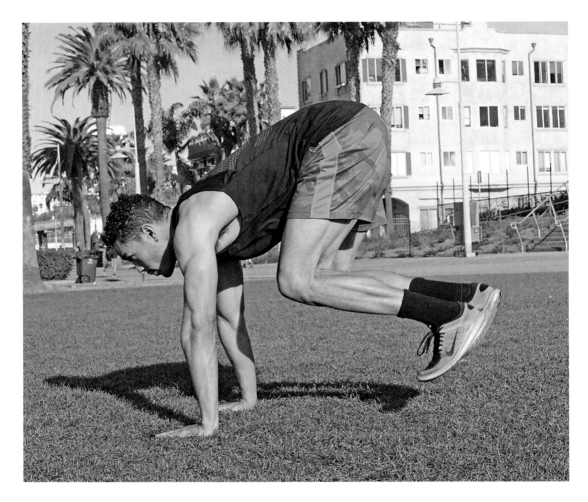

PLANK JUMPS

› Get into a plank position, then jump your feet forward as far as possible toward your hands.

› Jump back immediately and repeat.

ROCKING PLANKS

› Get into a forearm plank position, then shift your weight over your shoulders and then back again.

› Keep going back and forth for time.

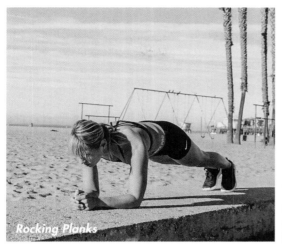

Rocking Planks

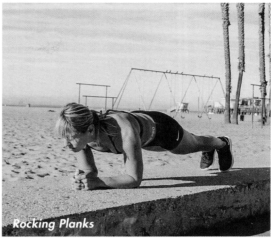

Rocking Planks

HOLLOW-BODY HOLDS FOR A STRONG, UNBREAKABLE BODY

Unless you grew up as a gymnast or have done a few CrossFit classes, you've probably never heard of the hollow-body position. This core strengthening exercise may feel strange when you first try it, but it's one of the most important fundamentals to learn in gymnastics and calisthenics movements.

Perfecting the hollow-body position will not only help protect your back and build a rock-solid core but it will also help make your body one strong, unbreakable line in all other movements. It's the position you should aim for when doing a countless number of exercises, from handstands to pull-ups and even double-unders.

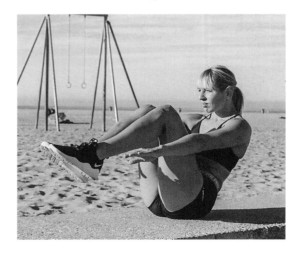

BENT-KNEE HOLLOW-BODY HOLD

This is the first variation of hollow-body hold and one you should perfect before moving onto more advanced versions.

> Lie down with your arms and legs extended. Engage your core,

thinking about pulling your belly button toward the floor.

› Slowly bend your knees as you reach your hands toward your feet, and hold.

MODIFIED HOLLOW-BODY HOLD

The next step in the hollow-body progression is to extend your legs.

› From the bent knee hollow-body position, slowly extend your legs until they're completely straight.

› Your ultimate goal should be to get them as close to the floor as possible, but start with the lowest position you can get to while still keeping your lower back in contact with the floor.

Work up to holding this position for three rounds of forty-five-second holds.

HOLLOW-BODY HOLD

The final hollow-body position is to have both your arms and legs extended.

› Extend both your arms and legs, thinking about keeping your core as tight as possible and your lower back pressed to the floor.

› Point your toes and extend your arms as you think about gluing them to your ears.

› Engage your entire body as you hold this position.

Work up to holding this position for three rounds of forty-five-second holds.

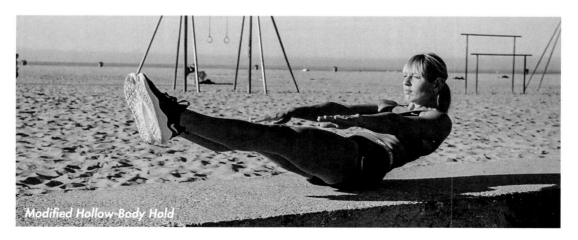

Modified Hollow-Body Hold

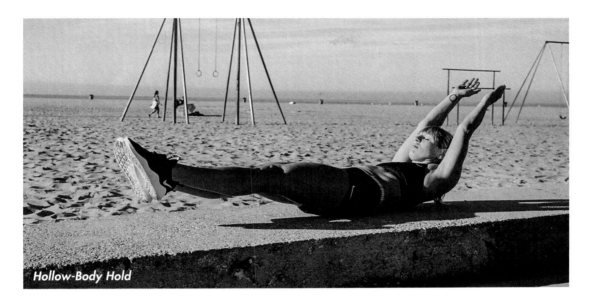

Hollow-Body Hold

HOLLOW-BODY ROCKS

Once you have a strong hollow-body hold, you can try hollow-body rocks to further strengthen the position and add variety to your workouts.

› From the full hollow-body position, begin to rock slowly back and forth.
› As you rock, you should think about not letting the position break at any time.

Work up to three rounds of sixty rocks.

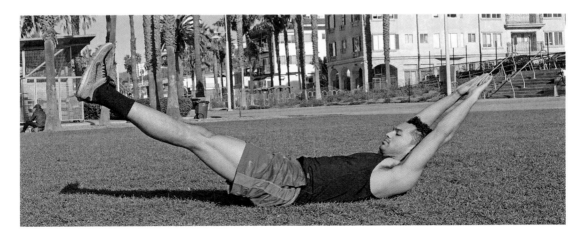

L-SITS FOR CORE STRENGTH

L-sits are one of those exercises that look a lot easier than they are. I mean really, holding your own legs out in front of you can't really be *that* hard, can it?

Yes, it can be.

The first time I tried to hold an L-sit, I thought that maybe my legs were too long, making it physically impossible for me to do an L-sit. Looking back now, it's pretty obvious I just didn't have the core or hip flexor strength to do one yet, but I didn't know that at the time.

L-sits require an immense amount of core strength, hip flexor strength, as well as shoulder and arm strength and hamstring flexibility. Just like with any more advanced exercises, work the following progressions and you'll be able to do the full thing in time.

> Note: L-sits can be performed on many different pieces of equipment, including parallel bars, parallettes, yoga blocks, hanging from a pull-up bar, or even on the ground. When first starting out, it's recommended to use parallel bars or something similar to work up to building strength.

TUCK L-SITS

› Grab on to parallel bars with both hands, squeeze your core, and push up through your shoulders.
› Tuck your knees toward your chest and hold for time.

Work up to holding this position for three thirty-second holds.

ONE-LEGGED L-SITS

› Grab on to parallel bars with both hands, squeeze your core, and push up through your shoulders.
› Tuck your knees toward your chest.

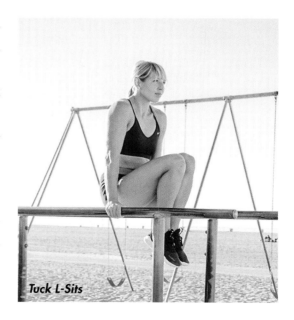
Tuck L-Sits

› Next, extend one leg out in front of you and hold for time.
› Make sure to work both sides.

Work up to holding this position for three thirty-second holds.

FULL L-SITS

› Grab on to parallel bars with both hands, squeeze your core, then extend both legs in front of you.
› Keep your legs as straight as possible in this position, focusing on keeping your chest up and toes pointed. Hold for time.

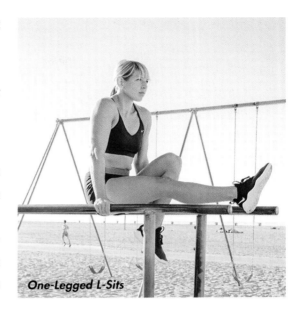

One-Legged L-Sits

Work up to holding this position for three thirty-second holds.

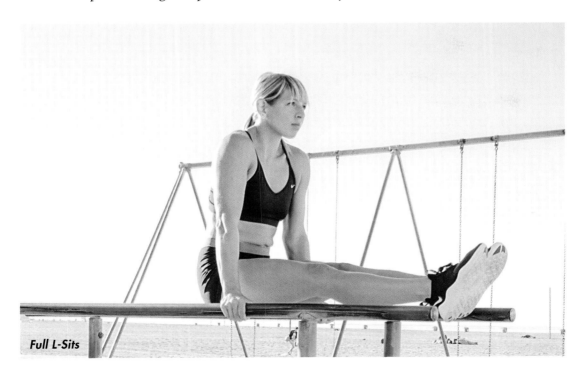

Full L-Sits

OTHER L-SIT VARIATIONS AND SUPPLEMENTAL EXERCISES

L-SIT TUCKS

> Get into a full L-sit position, tuck your knees toward your chest, and pause.

> Extend your legs back to the starting position.

> That's one rep.

PARALLEL BAR SCISSORS

> Start in a full L-sit position.

> Scissor your legs sideways, moving your right leg underneath your left leg, then alternate.

HIP FLEXOR TRIANGLES

Remember those hip flexor triangles from the pistol squat section (see page 53)? If you're having trouble holding your legs up during an L-sit, those can work wonders here, too. Aim for three sets of ten to fifteen hip flexor triangles per leg.

LEG RAISES AND OTHER PULL-UP BAR CORE EXERCISES

Adding pull-up bar-centered core exercises to your training can really help bring your core strength to the next level. As an added bonus, bar exercises like the ones in the next few pages are what will really help you get the six-pack (or eight-pack) you've always wanted!

HANGING KNEE RAISES

Grab a pull-up bar with your palms facing away from you and your hands about shoulder width apart. Ideally, the bar will be high enough that your feet clear the ground, but you can still do these if you have a low bar or a doorway bar—they'll just be a little more awkward.

> Pull your shoulders back and down while you tighten the rest of your body into a straight line.

> Keeping your legs tight together, tuck your knees up toward your chest while pointing your toes.

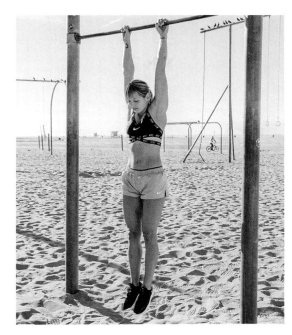
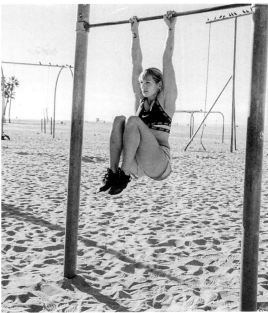

> Pause, then lower your legs back down into a straight line.

If you can't keep your knees completely together or you need to use some mo-

mentum to bring your legs up, that's okay for now. Eventually you'll want to be able to do knee raises without using any momentum at all.

Work up to three sets of ten reps.

HANGING LEG RAISES

> Grab a pull-up bar with both hands, pull your shoulders down and back, and tighten your core.

> Trying not to use momentum, raise your legs up until they're parallel to the floor, keeping them as straight as possible as you do so.

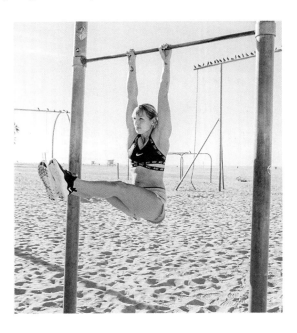

› Pause briefly, then lower back to the starting position. Don't forget to breathe!

Going from hanging knee tucks to hanging leg raises is a big jump, so don't get discouraged if you can't keep your legs completely straight or need to use a little momentum to help you up at the beginning. Over time, you'll be able to do these without using any momentum at all. Like always, it just takes time and practice.

Work up to three sets of ten reps.

KNEES TO ELBOWS

› Hang from a pull-up bar with your legs straight.
› Engage your core as you curl your knees up until they touch your elbows. Your knees will be turned out slightly rather than in a strict tuck.
› Try to use as little momentum as possible. Work up to three sets of ten reps.

TOES TO BAR

› Hang from a pull-up bar with straight legs and make sure everything is tight and your legs are locked together.

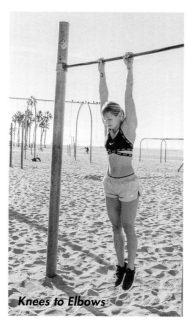
Knees to Elbows

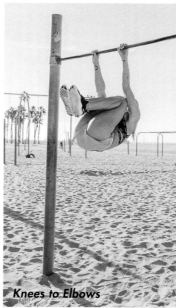
Knees to Elbows

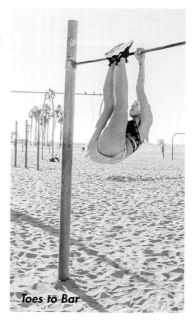
Toes to Bar

> Point your toes, raise them up to the bar, pause briefly, then lower down with control.

Eventually you'll want to be able to do these with completely straight legs, pointed toes, and using no momentum at all.

> Work up to three sets of ten reps.

OTHER PULL-UP BAR CORE EXERCISES
TWISTED HANGING KNEE RAISES

> Hang from a pull-up bar, bend your knees and lift them up toward your chest on one side.
> Lower back to the starting position, then twist up toward the opposite side.

TWISTED HANGING LEG RAISES

> Hang from a pull-up bar, then, keeping your legs as straight as you can, raise them up so that your feet touch the outside of your right hand.
> Lower down, then repeat on the left side. Each side is one rep.

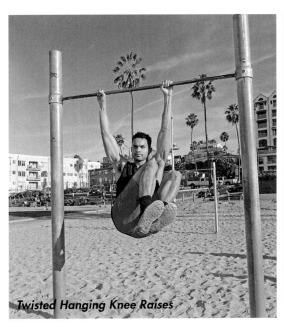
Twisted Hanging Knee Raises

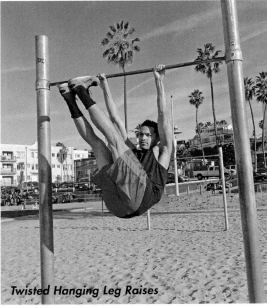
Twisted Hanging Leg Raises

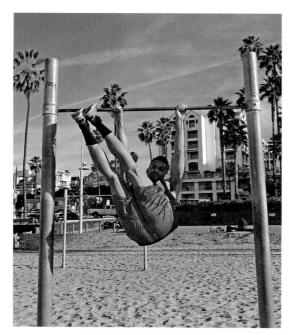
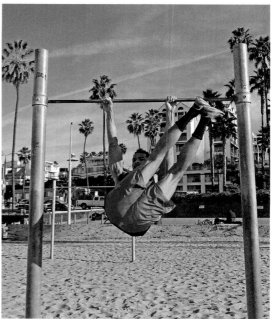

WINDSHIELD WIPERS

› Hang from a pull-up bar, then, keeping your legs as straight as you can, raise them up so that your feet touch the outside of your right hand.

› Without lowering down, rotate your legs to the left. Keep going back and forth without lowering down.

BRIDGES FOR A BULLETPROOF BACK

SHORT BRIDGES

Short bridges are great for beginners or people with previous back injuries. They gently work your back, glutes, and hamstring muscles.

› Lie on your back with your knees bent.

› Squeeze your glutes and keep your core tight as you raise your butt and hips as high as you can while still keeping your shoulders on the ground.

› Hold briefly, then lower down.

Work up to two sets of twenty reps.

FEET-ELEVATED BRIDGES

Feet-elevated bridges are the next step to help you ease into doing full bridges. These really start to work your shoulders as well as your back, butt, and leg muscles, and are the first step to getting really flexible and opening up your shoulders in a full bridge.

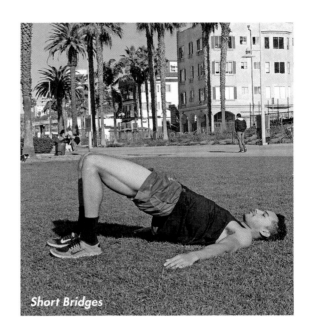

Short Bridges

Even if you can already do a floor bridge, feet-elevated bridges are a phenomenal way to open up your shoulders even more. I almost always include them as part of my clients' and my own warm-ups before going into floor bridges.

› Sit in front of a bench, a couple of steps, or a sturdy elevated surface that's about knee height.

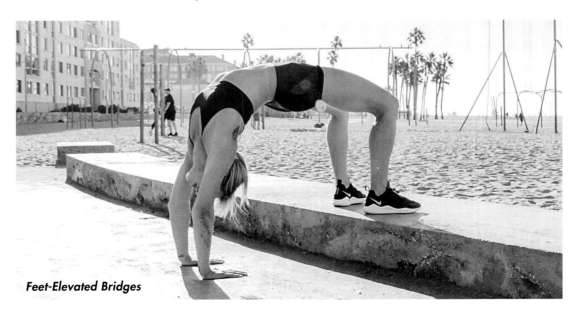

Feet-Elevated Bridges

> Place your feet on the bench, then place your hands by your head with your fingers pointing toward your feet.
> Try to push deep through your shoulders as you raise your hips as high as you can while keeping your arms straight. Remember to breathe.

Your eventual goal in this position is to stack your shoulders directly over your hands. Work toward three thirty-second holds.

FULL BRIDGES

> Lie on your back on the floor with your knees bent and your palms facing down by the sides of your head, fingers pointing toward your toes.
> Push your hips up as you squeeze your glutes, core, and leg muscles and push as much as possible through your shoulders.
> Look at your fingertips. Breathe.

Work toward three thirty-second holds.

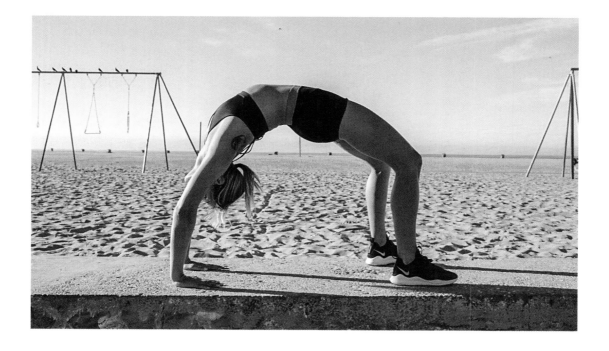

BRIDGE WALK-DOWNS

Bridge walk-downs are the first step in the progression toward stand-to-stand bridges. They can be a little scary at first, but you'll soon learn to trust yourself enough to know that you won't fall.

> Stand a few feet from a wall with your back facing toward the wall. The exact distance will depend on your height, so be prepared to experiment a bit.

> With your arms straight above you, lean backward, arching your back and squeezing your butt until your hands touch the wall, all the while looking at your hands.

> Slowly walk your hands down the wall as far as you can. Your goal should be to reach the ground to get into a full bridge.

> Once you reach the ground, simply sit down and stand back up.

Work toward two sets of five reps.

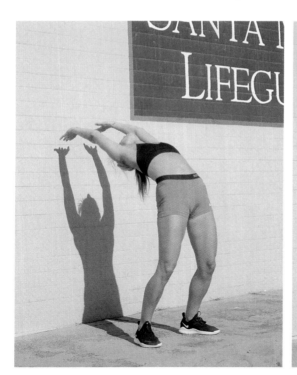
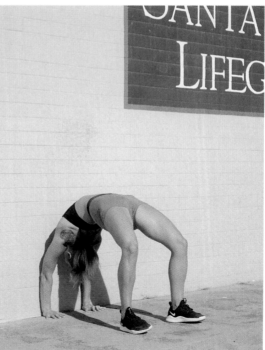

BRIDGE WALK-UPS

Bridge walk ups are significantly harder than walk downs, so don't get too discouraged the first time you try them. Walk-ups are a necessary step in training for stand-to-stand bridges. Once you get to this level, you'll be well on your way to a back of steel!

› Walk down the wall until you reach a full bridge.

› Once you get there, pause briefly, then use your hands to walk back up the wall, squeezing your butt and pushing your hips slightly forward as you stand up again.

› The more you practice this, the less you'll need to actually use your hands to help you stand back up.

Ultimately, you'll want to work toward not using your hands at all on the way up. Work toward two sets of five reps before moving on.

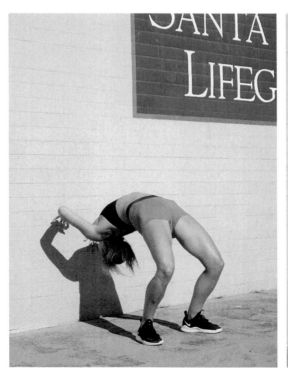
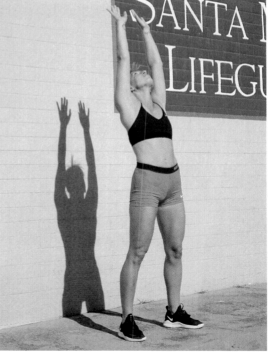

STAND-TO-STAND BRIDGES

Stand-to-stand bridges are the ultimate test of back strength and flexibility. If you can do even one, you're a total badass. If you can do ten in a row—you're amazing. You should be fairly comfortable with bridge walk-downs/ups before even attempting stand-to-stand bridges.

Once you have the necessary strength and flexibility for it, by far the most challenging part of a stand-to-stand bridge for most people is lowering into a bridge position from standing. If this is too daunting at first, try putting a pillow under where you might fall or at least make sure you're on a soft surface (*please* don't try these on concrete the first time).

> Look behind you as you lower down into a bridge with as much control as possible, pushing through your shoulders once you get there.

> Next comes the hard part: getting back up. Squeeze your glutes and tighten your core as you think about propelling your hips forward to help you stand up.

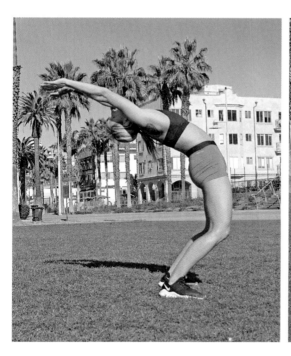 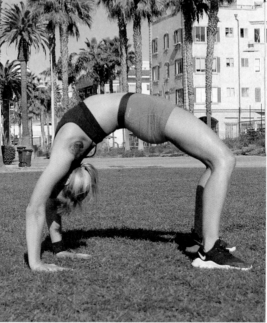

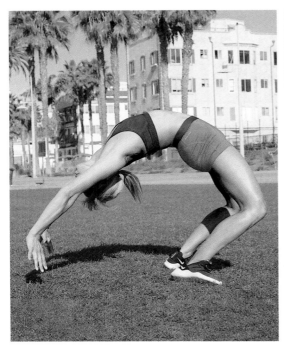 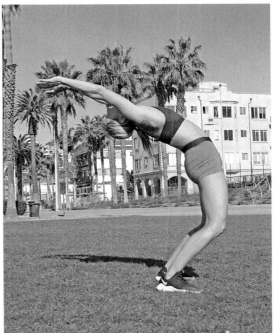

> It may help to rock slowly at first and use the momentum to help get you past the sticking point.

Work toward five solid reps.

MORE EXERCISES TO STRENGTHEN YOUR LOWER BACK

If you're having trouble with bridges or just want additional exercises to strengthen your lower back, glutes, and core, here are several worthwhile exercises you can do for that very purpose.

CANDLESTICK HIP BRIDGES

> Lie down on your back with your knees bent and feet on the floor.
> Raise one leg up straight above you, engage your core, then lift your hips up as high as you can while you squeeze your glutes.
> Lower down, making sure to work both sides.

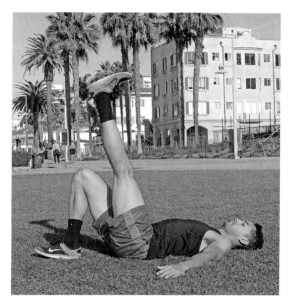 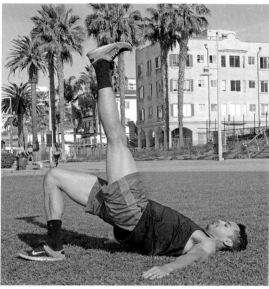

BIRD DOG

› Kneel with your elbows below your shoulders, chin tucked in, and neck long.

› Tuck your toes under, then extend one leg and opposite arm. You should feel your glutes working in the extended leg.

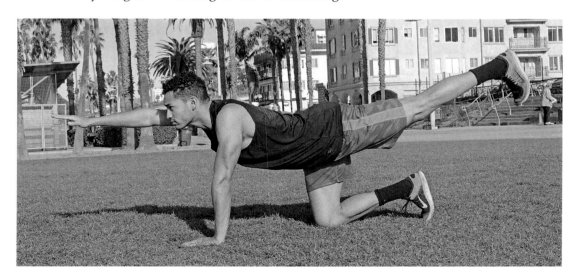

> When you feel the muscles in your lower back start to engage, you've gone high enough.
> Lower down, making sure to work both sides.

SUPERMAN HOLDS

> Lie on your stomach with your arms straight in front of you by your ears.
> Lift your arms and your legs simultaneously. Your arms should be straight and glued to your ears, as high up as you can get them. Your butt should be squeezed as hard as you can and your toes lifted off the floor.
> Try to focus on keeping your legs together as much as possible as you hold this position.

SUPERMAN RAISES

> Lie on the floor, then raise up to a superman position, keeping your legs as close together as you can.
> Pause, then lower back down.

SUPERMAN ROCKS

> Get into a superman position, then use your hips to rock back, making your feet raise higher in the air.

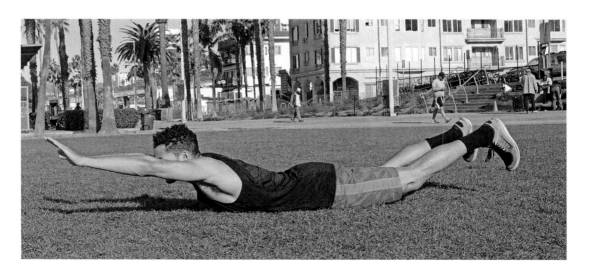

› Immediately pull your shoulders back and your hands upward so that your upper body rises while your feet fall closer to the floor.

› Focus on squeezing your glutes and using your hips for momentum. Never let your hands or feet touch the floor.

KICKOVERS

› Get into a full bridge, then rock forward so that you're pushing through your shoulders as far as you can.

› At the farthest point of the push, use the same leg you use to kick up into a handstand to kick as hard as you can and kick yourself over.

› You should aim to land on both feet, and, in true gymnastics style, with your hands straight up by your ears.

ADDITIONAL EQUIPMENT-FREE CORE EXERCISES

The following exercises can be done with zero equipment, so no matter where you are, you can still work your core. They're a great way to challenge yourself and add variety to your workouts.

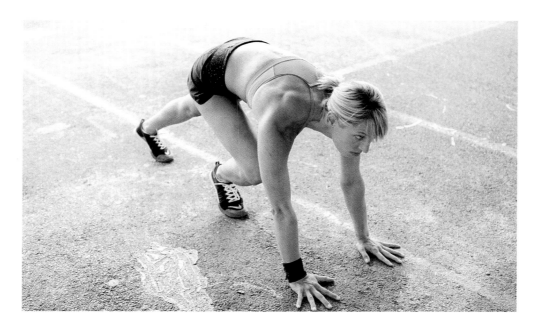

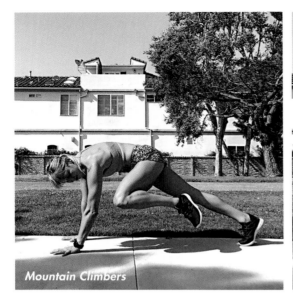
Mountain Climbers

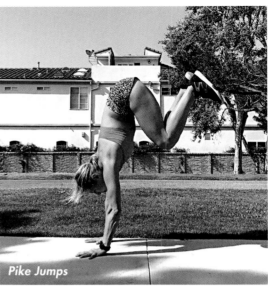
Pike Jumps

MOUNTAIN CLIMBERS

› Get in a plank position with your shoulders directly over your hands.

› Push up through your shoulders and engage your core.

› Bring one knee forward as if you were stepping toward your hand on the same side.

› Return it to the starting plank position as you simultaneously raise the other leg and bring it to your hand on the same side. Think about keeping your core tight and not letting your hips sag.

Once you get the hang of the movement, go for speed.

PIKE JUMPS

› Start in a downward dog position with your hands on the floor in front of you about shoulder-width apart.

› Jump your feet up as far as possible and land on one side.

› Trying not to pause, immediately jump to the other side and repeat.

SIDE PLANKS

› Get into a low plank position as you push through your shoulders and engage your core.

› Tip your body to one side so that you're balancing on one elbow and your feet are stacked on top of each other or directly next to one another.

› Pull your core in and make sure your hips aren't sagging.

To add an additional challenge to this exercise, try dipping toward the floor then back up, or extend your top leg up in a star position and hold.

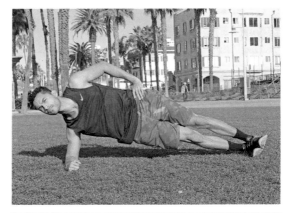

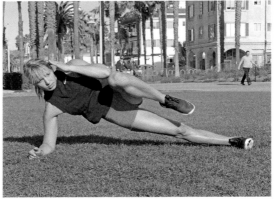

SIDE PLANKS WITH CRUNCH

› Get into a side plank position.

› Without dipping your hips, bring your top elbow and your right knee as close together as possible.

› Return to the starting position. Work both sides.

SIT-UPS

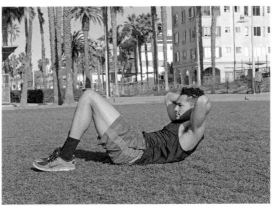

› Lie on the ground with your knees bent and your hands clasping the back of your head.

› Focus on keeping your core tight and pulled toward the ground as you use your core muscles to pull yourself up toward your knees.

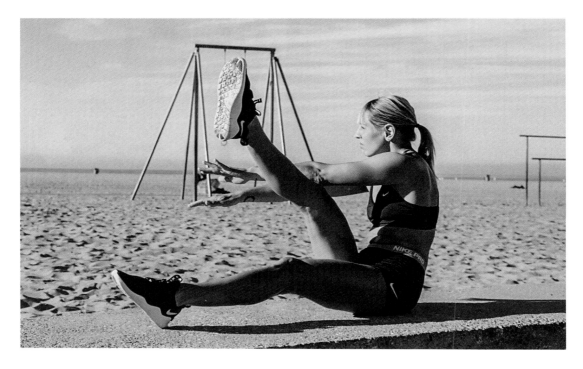

SPLIT LEG V-UPS

› Get into a hollow body position with your legs and arms extended.

› Lengthen as much as possible, then reach one arm toward your opposite foot, while keeping your leg straight.

› Lower back down and repeat on the other side.

STRAIGHT LEG SIT-UPS

› Lie on the ground with your legs straight and your hands clasped behind your head.

› Think about pointing your toes and keeping your legs tight and glued together.

› Use your core muscles to pull yourself up.

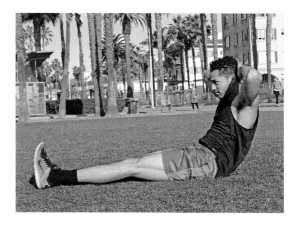

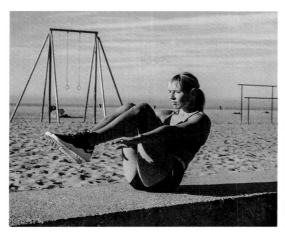
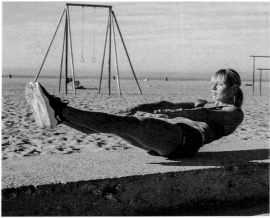

V-UP IN/OUTS

› Get into a hollow body position with your legs and arms extended. Think about lengthening everything and becoming as long as possible.

› Curl up, and as you do so, bend your knees toward your chest and reach toward your toes. Focus on keeping your knees tight together and abs pulled in as you reach forward.

› Lower back down to the starting position with control.

V-UPS

› Get into a hollow body position with your legs and arms extended.

› Lengthen as much as possible, then curl your arms and legs up into a V position, touching your toes if possible.

› Try to keep everything straight and tight as you squeeze your core and reach for your toes.

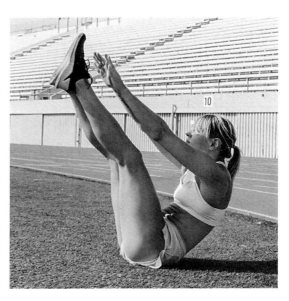

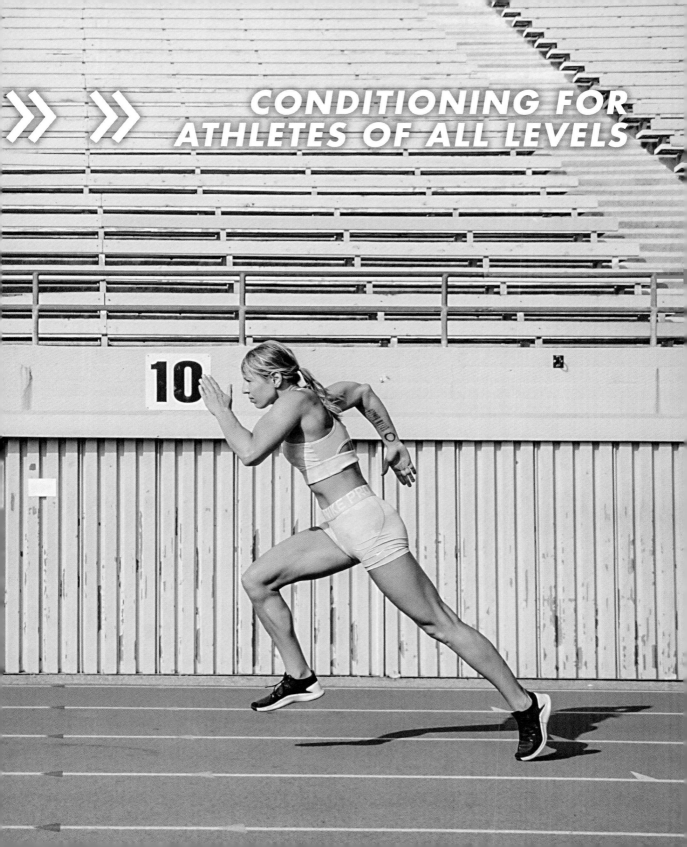

CONDITIONING FOR
ATHLETES OF ALL LEVELS

BURPEES: WHY THEY SHOULD BE YOUR FAVORITE EXERCISE

Burpees are one of those exercises that people absolutely love to hate but are catching on in popularity due to the amazing amount of awesome benefits they provide.

Here are five reasons why burpees should be your favorite exercise ever:

1. BURPEES MAKE YOUR BODY A FAT-BURNING MACHINE.

Since burpees are an intense full-body exercise, they burn a ton of calories. Better yet, they speed up your metabolism throughout the day—meaning you'll burn more calories all day long, even after you're long done with your burpees. So, if you want to lose weight, ditch the recumbent bike and elliptical machine and do some burpees instead.

2. THEY MAKE YOU STRONGER.

Burpees are a full-body strength training exercise and the ultimate example of functional fitness. With every rep, you'll work your arms, chest, quads, glutes, hamstrings, and core muscles. After a few sets of burpees, your legs should feel a little bit like lead.

3. THEY'RE A GREAT CONDITIONING TOOL.

Burpees are one of the best exercises for developing conditioning and endurance. Whether your goal is to learn a new sport, train for a triathlon, hike a big mountain, or, just to look good, burpees should be a part of your regular workout routine.

4. THEY'RE PORTABLE AND REQUIRE NO EQUIPMENT.

The best thing about burpees? They require absolutely no equipment. You can do burpees in your house, in a nearby park, or even in your hotel room.

5. YOU CAN ADD THEM TO ALMOST ANY WORKOUT.

Burpees are fast-paced, dynamic, and never boring. They're perfect for HIIT training or as a stand-alone exercise. Just try doing a hundred burpees in a row for time (no, really, try it) and you'll see what I mean.

HOW TO DO A BURPEE

There are certain trainers and fitness enthusiasts who will tell you there's only one way to do a burpee—because while burpees are a pretty simple exercise, they're also one that people get really opinionated about. Yet, just like with any other exercise, there are many different ways to do burpees, and different benefits for each type.

To be honest, I don't really care which variety of burpee you do, as long as you're working hard and challenging yourself. These are the most common burpee variations:

BURPEE WITH A FULL PUSH-UP
› From standing, drop down to a push-up position and do a full push-up.
› Immediately jump your feet toward your hands.
› Jump straight up, adding a clap for pizazz at the very top.

PLANK-STYLE BURPEES
› Start from standing, then drop down into a high plank position before jumping your feet back toward your hands and jumping straight up in the air.
› Keep your core tight and glutes engaged.

CHEST-TO-FLOOR BURPEES
You've probably seen this style of burpee most often in CrossFit gyms or MMA training, and this is the one that inspires the most controversy.
› Squat down from standing, place your hands on the floor, then kick your feet back quickly and land so that your chest hits the floor.
› Rather than doing a full push-up, bow your chest up, jump your feet back toward your hands, then jump up and get some air.
› Think about keeping your core and glutes tight the entire time.
In case you're wondering: no, this style of burpee won't automatically hurt your back—your back is *made* to bend this way. However, if you have previous back issues, plank-style burpees or burpees with a push-up are your safest option.

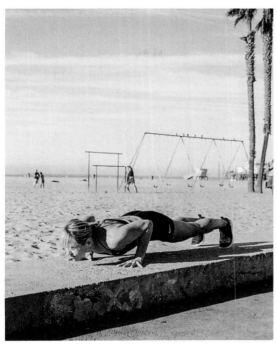
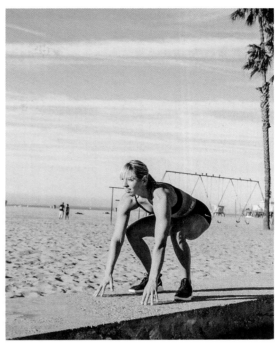
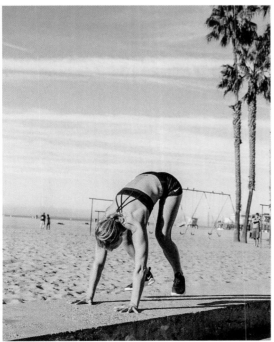
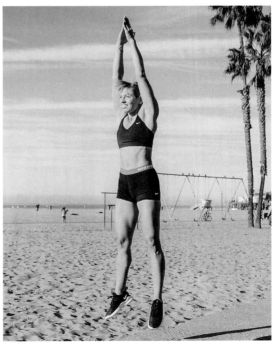

OTHER COOL BURPEE VARIATIONS

If regular burpees somehow aren't enough for you or if you just want to mix it up here and there, there are several cool different burpee variations you can try:

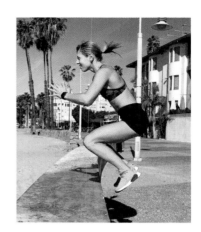

BURPEE BOX JUMPS

›   Get in front of a plyo box or sturdy elevated surface, do a burpee, then rather than jump straight up, jump up onto the box.

›   Jump or step down from the box and immediately do another burpee.

BURPEE LATERAL JUMPS

›   Drop down and do a burpee and instead of the jump up, jump as far as you can to one side.

›   Immediately do another burpee, then jump back to the starting position.

BURPEE PULL-UPS

›   Get in front of a pull-up bar and do a regular burpee. Instead of clapping on the way up, jump up and do a pull-up.

›   Lower down and repeat.

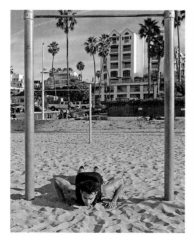
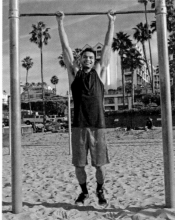
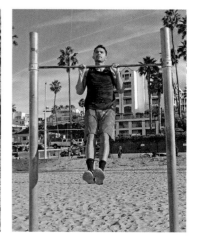

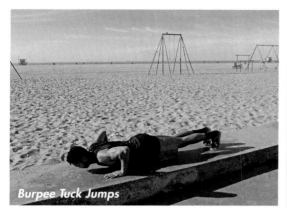
Burpee Tuck Jumps

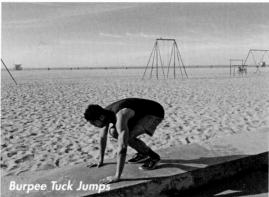
Burpee Tuck Jumps

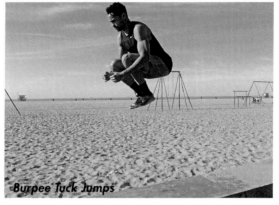
Burpee Tuck Jumps

BURPEE STEP-OVERS

› Stand to the side of a plyo box or a sturdy elevated surface.

› Do a burpee, then step onto the box with one leg, then bring the other leg up so that you're standing on top of the box.

› Step down with one leg, then bring the other leg down to the ground and immediately do another burpee.

BURPEE TUCK JUMPS

› Do a full burpee, but instead of the clapping jump on the way up, do a tuck jump instead.

› Focus on keeping your knees close together and tight toward your chest as you jump.

MOUNTAIN CLIMBER BURPEES

› Drop down into a plank and immediately do four mountain climbers, two on each side.

› Jump up explosively, reaching your hands toward the sky.

› Return to the starting position and repeat.

PLYOMETRIC LOWER-BODY EXERCISES

If you want to take your conditioning to the next level, there's no better way to do so than to add in plyometric training to your workouts.

Plyometric exercises (or plyos for short) are quick, powerful exercises that are performed in a short amount of time to help you build speed and power. They're an essential part of every athlete's training—and you're no different!

WHY YOU SHOULD DO PLYOMETRICS REGULARLY

- **They get your heart rate up quickly.** Getting your heart rate up fast is one of the main benefits of HIIT training. By doing plyos regularly, you'll be working to build a stronger, healthier heart.
- **They make your body a fat-burning machine.** Not only will you be burning more fat during your plyometric workout but the afterburn effect of plyometric training means that your body will be a fat burning machine twenty-four to forty-eight hours after you've finished your workout.
- **They'll help boost your athletic performance.** Plyos can help you improve your athletic performance for nearly any sport, whether it's basketball, boxing, MMA, soccer, or any ball-related sport. Even long-distance runners can benefit from plyometric training because they often need to sprint during the last stretch of their race. This is where having extra power can help tremendously.
- **They build strength.** Working your plyos regularly will really help you to build up your explosive strength. You'll not only get faster; you'll build strength and explosiveness as well, all with just your own bodyweight.
- **They get results in less time.** If your goals include building

strength, getting faster, leaner, and becoming a more powerful athlete, then you should be doing plyos on a regular basis.

The best part is that you can get all of this done in a relatively short amount of time. Since plyometric training demands a lot of energy from your body, it'll be over before you know it.

Here are some of the most effective lower-body exercises you can do to take your lower-body training to the next level:

BOX JUMPS

Box jumps have a number of benefits, including increasing your speed, coordination, vertical leap, and overall athleticism.

If you're brand-new to box jumps, you may need to first build up your confidence and assure your mind that you can, in fact, jump with two feet onto a higher surface.

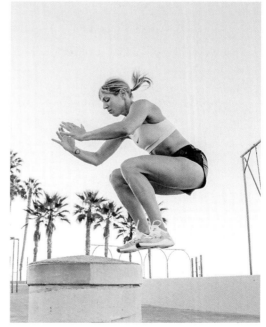

› Stand in front of a plyo box or a sturdy elevated surface, bend your knees slightly, and then jump onto the box.

› Land on top of the box with both feet, straighten your legs slightly, then step or jump back down.

If the transition from the ground to the top of the box doesn't go as smoothly as you hope at first, don't be overly discouraged. Work at your own pace, be safe, and you'll get faster and more coordinated with time. Start with a smaller plyo box or a sturdy elevated surface, and slowly increase the height as your jumping improves.

To build maximum explosiveness with box jumps, try to work toward not pausing in between jumps.

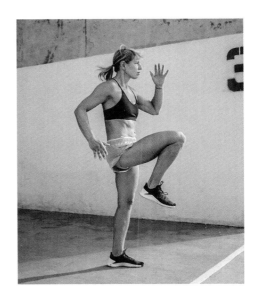

HIGH KNEES

High knees will get you nearly the same benefits as sprinting—without having to go anywhere. As a result, they're a perfect conditioning exercise when you don't have a lot of space, and are a fantastic addition to any workout.

› Start by driving one knee toward your chest as high as you can.
› Immediately bring it to the ground and replace it with your other knee.

When you perform high knees, you should focus on keeping your body as tight as possible, keeping your core engaged and shoulders pulled back and down (instead of up to your ears) during the entire movement. Use your arms to pump you, just as you would if you were sprinting. Try to go as fast as you can while still keeping tight with good form.

CANDLESTICK JUMP-UPS

› From standing, squat down, roll onto your back, and lift your legs off the floor straight above you in a candlestick position.
› Try to keep your knees as straight as possible and your toes pointed as you contract your abs.
› Bend your knees and quickly lower them to the ground, touching or almost touching your butt.
› Use momentum from the roll and lean forward and stand up.
› Immediately jump into the air with your arms reaching toward the sky, then repeat.

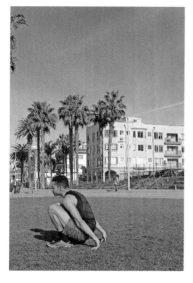 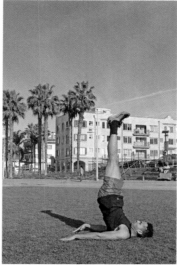 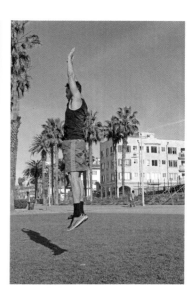

JUMP LUNGES

› Start in a lunge position with your back knee a few inches from the floor.

› Jump up explosively and switch legs so that your rear leg is in the front and front leg is in the rear.

› Repeat on the other side.

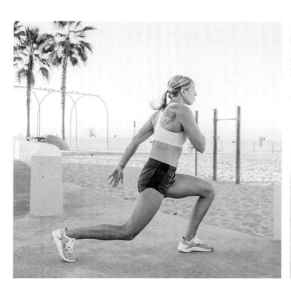 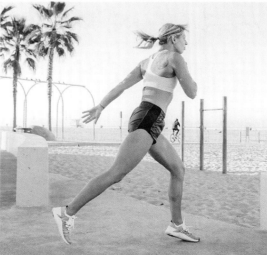

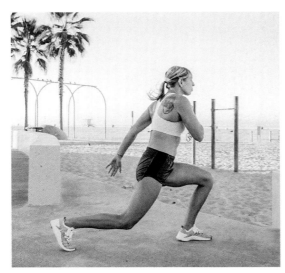 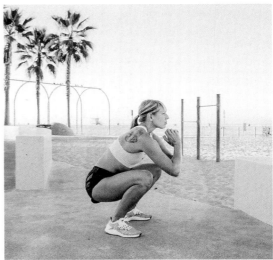

JUMP LUNGE SQUAT COMBO

› Start in a lunge position with your back knee a few inches from the floor.
› Jump up explosively and switch legs so that your rear leg is in the front and front leg is in the rear. Repeat with the other leg.
› Jump back up, but this time, land in a squat position.
› Jump up and repeat the sequence.

LONG JUMPS

› Stand with your feet hip-width apart.
› Bend your knees and jump explosively as far forward as you can, using your arms for momentum.

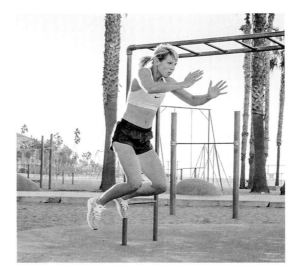

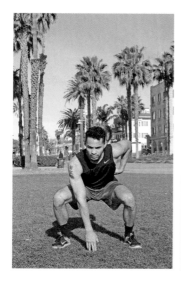
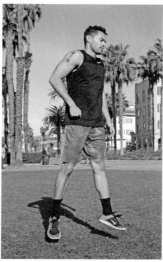

SNOWBOARDER JUMPS

› Stand with your feet about hip-width apart, then squat down to about parallel.

› Jump up explosively as you turn 180 degrees in midair.

› Land back in a squat position, then repeat going in the opposite direction.

SQUAT JUMPS

› Stand with your feet about hip-width apart, then squat down to about parallel.

› Jump up as explosively as you can while using your arms for momentum, landing back in a squat.

› Immediately jump up again without pausing.

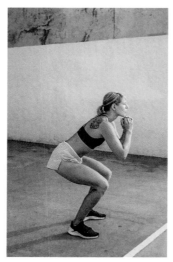
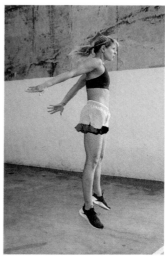

TUCK JUMPS

› Stand with your feet about hip-width apart, then jump up as high as you can, tucking your knees into your chest as you do so.

› Land and repeat as fast as you can, trying not to pause in between each jump.

There are countless variations of the above plyometric exercises. In fact, you can make nearly any bodyweight exercise a plyometric exercise by adding dynamic movement to it. Get creative, and have fun with it!

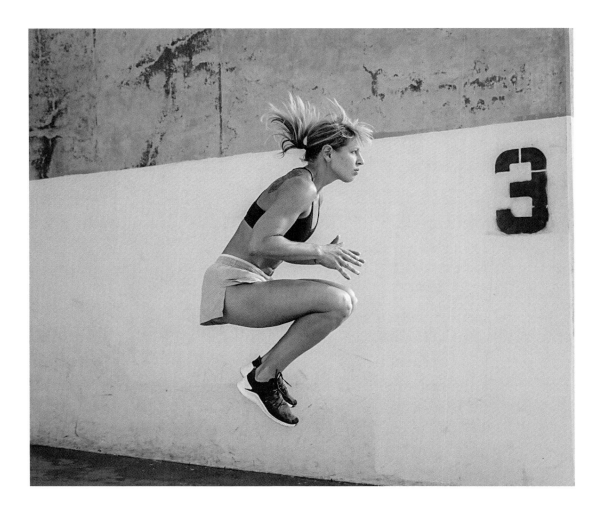

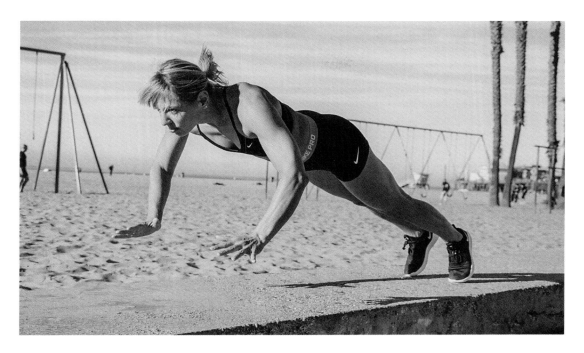

PLYOMETRIC UPPER-BODY EXERCISES

The first thing that comes to mind when most people think of plyometric exercises are lower-body exercises like squat jumps and jump lunges. Yet there are plenty of ways to make upper-body exercises plyometric as well. Working the following plyometric push-up variations are an awesome way to build power and explosiveness, and are especially useful for sports such as boxing or any combat sports, basketball, tennis, or any sport requiring a good amount of upper-body power.

Here are some of the most effective lower-body exercises you can do to kick your upper-body conditioning up a notch.

PUSH-UPS WITH FLOOR PUSH-OFF

This is the easiest explosive push-up variation and the one you should start with if you've never tried them before.

› Get into a push-up position, tighten your core, and push up through your shoulders.

› Bend your arms into a half push-up—no need to go all the way down on these—and then on the way up, push up explosively so that your hands leave the ground. Even just a tiny bit of air counts.

If this is too hard right now, you can make this easier by placing your hands on an elevated surface, such as a couch or even a countertop.

PUSH-UP HOPS

› Follow the form for the previous variation, except this time jump up with your feet as well.

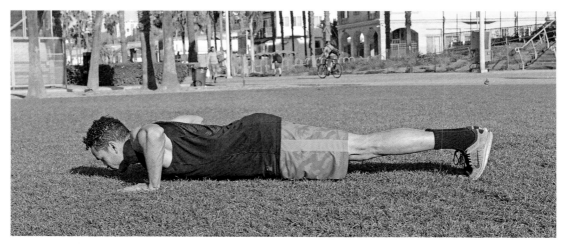

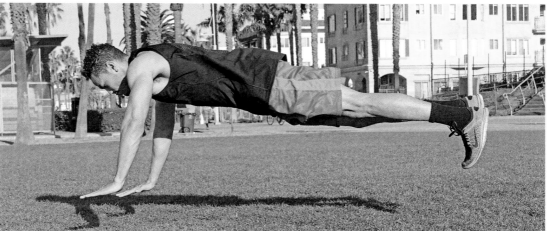

› This explosive push-up variation does take more coordination but because your legs are naturally more powerful than your arms, it takes less strength.

HANDS-ELEVATED CLAPPING PUSH-UPS

› Place your hands on a box, bench, or a pile of mats and get into a push-up position, keeping your core tight.

› Bend your arms into a half push-up, then as you're coming back up, push up explosively so that your hands leave the bench for a short moment.

The lower the surface, the more challenging these will be.

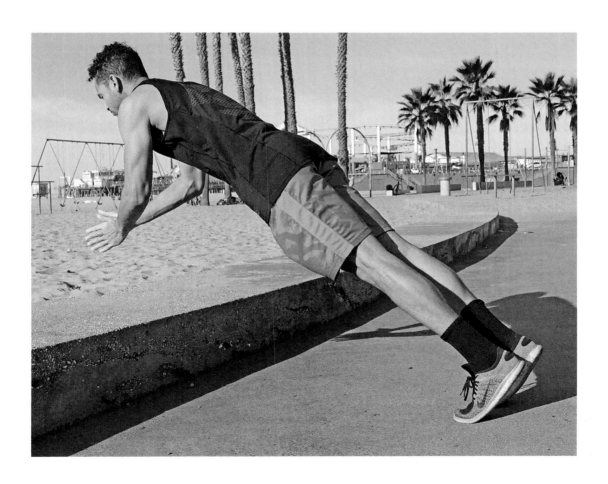

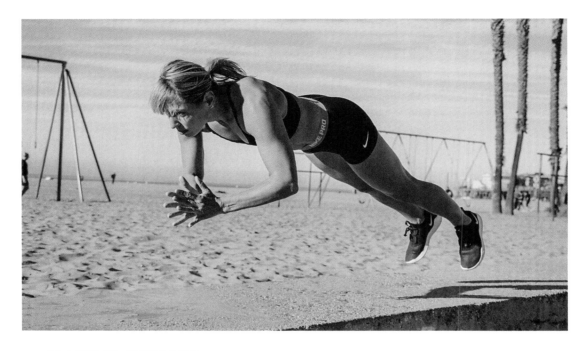

CLAPPING PUSH-UPS

These are the same as the hands-elevated version except that you'll be doing them on the floor.

If you're nervous about falling on your face, try doing them on a softer surface like a gym mat or grass.

OTHER PLYOMETRIC PUSH-UP VARIATIONS

Once you can do around ten or more clapping push-ups in a row, you can start getting more creative. Here are a few ideas of things to try if you're more advanced and looking for an extra challenge:

› Double clap at top of push-up
› Clap behind back
› Superman push-up

The possibilities are endless. As always, use your creativity and have fun with it.

JUMPING ROPE TO WHIP YOU INTO SHAPE

There's a reason why boxers and elite athletes embrace jumping rope as a consistent form of cardio and conditioning: it's a cheap, effective, and efficient way of getting—and staying—in shape fast.

If you haven't picked up a jump rope since you were a kid, you might be surprised at how difficult it is. Even if you're already in pretty good shape, jumping rope is a whole other animal, requiring strong legs, coordination, and a high Vo_2 max—that is, your body's ability to utilize oxygen during intense exercise. More likely than not, your calves will start to ache and you'll be breathing hard within just a few minutes of jumping rope.

But don't let this description intimidate you—a little jumping rope goes a long way. Jumping rope consistently will get you fit in a very short amount of time, especially if you're constantly challenging yourself to try more difficult variations.

Without a doubt, a jump rope will be the best eight to twenty dollars you've ever spent on fitness equipment. Not only does jumping rope take very little space to do but jump ropes are extremely portable, giving you an excuse-free method of getting your heart rate up anywhere you go.

CHOOSING THE CORRECT JUMP ROPE HEIGHT

Jumping with a rope that's either too short or too long for your height will make any jumping rope exercise significantly more difficult and less efficient.

Jump ropes are meant to be adjusted, and this is one of the first things you should do when you get a new rope. Doubled over, your jump rope should hit at about chest level (if you're more advanced it can be slightly shorter).

If your jump rope is too long, just tie a knot or two to shorten it.

There are several different jump rope variations you can include in your training to elevate your fitness and improve your coordination:

SINGLE-UNDERS

Single-unders are the most basic form of jumping rope and the one that you probably think of first when you think of jumping rope.

› Grab your jump rope with both hands, swing it in front of you, and then jump over it.

› Try to think about keeping everything as tight as possible as you jump.

› Your legs should be close together and you should actively engage your core muscles.

› You should also aim to keep your hands as close to your sides as possible, rather than flaring your elbows and arms out to the side.

> *Note: If you're substituting single-unders for double-unders in one of the workouts later on in this book, you'll need to do three single-unders for every double under.*

DOUBLE-UNDERS

Double-unders have long been a drill embraced by boxers and other fighters. They're incredible for overall conditioning, coordination, and building endurance. And if you've ever done CrossFit, you've probably encountered them there, too.

While the concept of double-unders is simple—get the rope under your feet twice in a single jump—they require an incredible amount of speed, strength, and coordination to actually execute. Expect to spend weeks, maybe even months, before you get really good at them.

Feeling intimidated yet? Don't be. Yes, it will take time and practice, but in time you *will* be able to do them.

Here are a few things to keep in mind when practicing double-unders:

› TRY STARTING WITH A FEW SINGLE-UNDERS. It helps to start with a few single-unders first, *then* try for a double under or two.

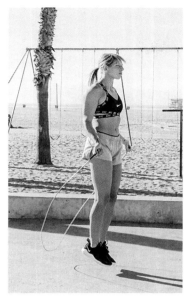 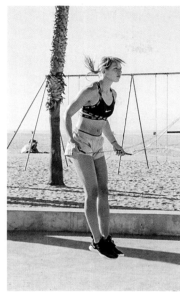 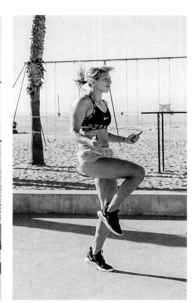

> › STAY TIGHT. Engage your core, and keep your legs tight together throughout the exercise. This will help with efficiency and control.
> › USE YOUR WRISTS. Keep your arms close to your body and use your wrists to spin the rope, not your arms. Fail to do this and your shoulders will fatigue quickly.
> › BEND YOUR KNEES AS LITTLE AS POSSIBLE. Try to keep your legs straight and your body in a hollow-body position, rather than bending your knees into more of a tuck jump. This is a much more efficient way to do double-unders and will help you fatigue less quickly.

Most of all, practice, practice, practice! You'll never get better at them unless you *try*.

HIGH KNEES USING A JUMP ROPE

Perform high knees while swinging a jump rope forward. This requires a greater degree of coordination than regular high knees, so don't be worried if you trip up (literally)—you'll catch on quickly.

As with the other jumping rope techniques, make sure to keep the rope nice and tight to your body rather than holding your arms out away from you. This will help you focus on driving your knees up as quickly as possible without overly fatiguing your shoulders.

OTHER COOL JUMP ROPE VARIATIONS TO TRY

Once you master the basics, you can start to get more creative with your jumping rope. Here are a few fun tricks to try.

CRISSCROSS ARMS
› Before each jump, bring your left hand to your right side and your right hand to your left side so that your arms are crossed.
› After you've made the first jump, resume your normal hands positioning to prepare for the next jump.

CRISSCROSS FEET
› Before each jump, cross your feet in front of each other.
› Resume your normal position for your next jump.
› Switch your starting foot each time.

FRONT-TO-BACK JUMPS
Jump forward and backward continuously while jumping over the rope.

SIDE-TO-SIDE JUMPS
Jump side to side continuously while jumping over the rope.

SIDE SWINGS
Twirl the rope to one side before jumping over the rope.

SINGLE-LEG JUMPS
Hold one leg up while you jump on the other leg.

SPRINTS FOR A LEAN, POWERFUL BODY

Although I'm personally not a huge fan of long-distance running, there's no question that sprints are one of the best exercises for building explosive power and boosting conditioning. They're also one of the best ways to shed fat and build a lean and powerful body.

And while they may seem fairly self-explanatory, there are actually several tips that will make your sprints more efficient and more powerful. Keep these in mind the next time you sprint.

› START WITH THE CORRECT FOOT FORWARD. Most right-handed people will want their left foot forward, and most left-handed people will want their right foot forward. Having the correct foot forward will lead to a more powerful start.

› EXPLODE OFF YOUR BACK FOOT WHEN STARTING YOUR SPRINT. This foot gives you the most power, which is why it also tends to be your strong side.

› AIM TO TOUCH THE GROUND ONLY WITH YOUR TOES AND THE BALL OF YOUR FOOT. Stay off your heels to be lighter and faster on your feet.

› RUN WITH A CIRCULAR MOTION. Think like a cyclist and move your feet in a circular motion, raising your thighs up until they are parallel to the ground, and driving your knees up and down (rather than an ovular or reaching-out motion).

› LEAN SLIGHTLY FORWARD AND ENGAGE YOUR CORE. Use gravity to your advantage by leaning your body slightly forward as you sprint. This will make each stride more efficient. Keep your core engaged the entire time.

› SHORTEN YOUR STRIDE. While it may seem counterintuitive, longer strides are less efficient and waste energy. Focus on short, quick strides for maximum efficiency and speed.

› KICK YOUR FEET TOWARD YOUR BUTT. As you push off from the forefoot and toes, bring your heels up toward your butt on each stride.

› SWING YOUR ARMS. Make an L shape with your arms. Pump your fists as high as your chin and your elbows back as far as possible for momentum.

› BREATHE! Relax into the sprint and try to sync your breathing toward the rhythm of your feet. This will help you reduce wasted energy from muscle tension.

› SPRINT SHORT DISTANCES. To maximize speed, you want to train only when you're at your fastest. That means you shouldn't aim to sprint for longer than twenty to thirty seconds in one burst. After about thirty seconds your effort will naturally decrease to more of a jog.

FIVE

THE WORKOUTS

*The only way to define your limits
is by going beyond them.*

—ARTHUR C. CLARKE

A lthough you can try the exercises in this book in whichever order you like, most people want to know how to put them together as efficiently as possible. The following eight-week plans are sample comprehensive programs to help you build your skill arsenal while helping you to get fitter, faster, and stronger in less time. They can be used as stand-alone plans or you can do them in addition to any sport-specific training, yoga, or other activities you enjoy.

I put these workouts together based on years of training experience with efficiency and maximum effectiveness in mind. The workouts are for athletes of all levels, so no matter where you're at on the spectrum, you *can* do them.

Before you get started, there are a few things you should know.

GETTING STARTED

First, you'll need to choose between the Athlete workout plan (three times a week) and the Super Athlete workout plan (five times a week). This is completely up to you and how often you want to train. If you're a total beginner, do a lot of other sports or activities on top of the workouts, or are just insanely busy, you'll most likely want to choose the Athlete plan. On the other hand, if you're looking to really push your strength and conditioning levels to the next level and you have the time and energy to do so, go for the Super Athlete plan.

Either way, I strongly recommend that active people take at least one (if not two) full days off from strenuous exercise per week. This is not an option. Giving your body the proper amount of rest allows it to recover and grow stronger and fitter than before. Without proper recovery time, you'll most likely end up injured and overtrained and have to start back at step one all over again.

I know plenty of strong and capable athletes who have failed to take proper rest days and end up injured because of it. Don't do it.

But just because you take a day off from intense training doesn't mean you have to sit on the couch and not move all day long. Staying active will actually help you recover faster, and will also keep you in the habit of exercising and moving on a regular basis. Going for a leisurely bike ride, taking a long walk or an easy hike, or playing a friendly game of tennis with a friend are all totally acceptable active rest day activities.

PROGRESSING IN THE WORKOUTS

When you first look at the workouts, one of the things you'll probably notice right away is that the workout of the day notes the full, standard version of each exercise.

Since everyone who picks up a copy of this book is at a different level (and because, without actually talking to you and determining your goals, I can't know exactly what level you are personally at), the customization I would give if I were training you one-on-one is different from what I can give in this book. It didn't make sense to make a "beginner" level because one beginner may be able to do more advanced lower-body plyometric exercises but not full push-ups, while another beginner may be able to do the opposite.

So, before you look at the workouts and say "I can't do X exercise!" or "X exercise is too easy for me!" keep the following things in mind.

Do whichever progression of the exercise you're currently working on in the workouts. This means that if the workout of the day calls for pull-ups and you're currently working on jumping pull-ups, you should do jumping pull-ups in the workout. If the workout calls for push-ups and you're currently working on one-arm push-ups, you should do one-arm push-ups in the workout.

If at any point in the workout you fatigue and can no longer do the current progression of the exercise in the workout, immediately go to the easier progression—don't just give up or stop altogether. So, if you're doing push-ups and your strength gives out, switch to hands-elevated push-ups. This will keep you working hard and help you to continue to build strength and endurance, even when your muscles inevitably fail.

Most of all, work hard! These workouts are only effective if you give them absolutely everything you've got. Push yourself on a regular basis and you'll be amazed at what you can accomplish.

TRACKING YOUR PROGRESS

I highly recommend that you keep some sort of written (or digital) record of your workouts. Keeping a tracking log will help you stay motivated when at some point along the way you feel like giving up because it seems like you're going nowhere, even though you've actually made a great deal of progress. It will also give you something to look back on when you're feeling discouraged and want reassurance that you're not just wasting your time.

Ideally, your tracking log will include:

> Your workout for the day and what you did, including completed reps or relevant times
> How you felt during the workout, approximate length of breaks, etc.
> Any PRs (personal records) you achieved for the day
> Your mood/how motivated you were/any other relevant notes

Once you get the hang of doing this regularly, it's pretty cool to be able to look back on your earlier training notes and see just how far you've come.

EQUIPMENT

For both the Athlete workout plan and Super Athlete workout plan, the only equipment you'll need is an interval timer or app, a pull-up bar, a dip bar or parallel bars, a jump rope, and something to jump on (a sturdy set of stairs is just fine).

If you want to add even more of a challenge for some of the exercises, feel free to grab a set of dumbbells, a sandbag, or just fill a backpack with some heavy stuff and go to town.

INTENSITY IS KEY

If you've been exercising for a while, you probably already realize that what you get out of your workout is 100 percent based on what you put into it. If you work hard, you'll get stronger, fitter, faster, and become an overall better athlete. If you half-ass it . . . well, you'll get half-assed results.

That being said, there are a few different things you can do to make sure you put the maximum intensity into these workouts.

START WITH THE MOST DIFFICULT PROGRESSION YOU CAN DO

Whenever you're doing high-intensity exercises and workouts like the ones in this book, you should make sure you're doing the most challenging version of an exercise that you can do.

For example, if a workout includes push-ups and you can do at least two full push-ups with your hands on the floor (with good form)—start with full push-ups! Don't take the easier route and put your hands on an elevated surface just because you're worried you'll fatigue later in the workout. If you do fatigue and can no longer do an exercise with good form, then by all means go to the previous progression of the exercise—but only *after* you fatigue.

Starting out with the hardest version of the exercise will help you grow stronger, faster.

MINIMIZE YOUR REST TIMES

We've all seen those people in the gym who spend most of their gym session talking with their friends or checking out Instagram while "resting" in between sets. In reality this is mostly a waste of time, and leads to a long, inefficient workout.

The workouts in this book are designed with minimal rest to keep them as efficient as possible. You'll notice that most of the time an upper-body exercise is followed by a lower-body one (or a cardio exercise followed by a strength exercise, etc.)—this is on purpose so that a specific part of your body can rest while another part of your body works hard. This allows for maximum efficiency, meaning you'll get an entire workout done in less time.

That being said, if you do need a little extra rest, take it! Listen to your body and make sure to pay attention to form while continuously challenging yourself.

TRAIN LIKE I'M THERE RIGHT WITH YOU!

The main reasons that people hire personal trainers are not that they couldn't find a workout routine elsewhere but for the motivation, consistency, and in-person pressure.

Since you made it this far in this book, I'm guessing you already have much of the motivation and consistency, so now that you have the workouts, the last piece of the puzzle is to work out like I'm right there next to you, cheering you on.

There's no question about it, having a trainer or even a buddy there training next to you will often make you push harder than you would have otherwise. So, during these workouts, I want you to do everything you can do to act like this is the case. This will help keep you honest with yourself and working as hard as you possibly can.

YOU'VE GOT THIS!

YOUR EIGHT-WEEK PLAN TO GET FITTER, FASTER, AND STRONGER

The next section outlines an eight-week workout plan you can follow to get fitter, faster, and stronger than ever before. Before you start, you'll need to choose between the Athlete plan or the Super Athlete plan. Although which plan you choose is entirely up to you, there are good reasons to choose either one.

HERE'S WHY YOU MIGHT WANT TO CHOOSE THE ATHLETE PLAN:
› You don't have a lot of time each week to dedicate to your training
› You are new(ish) to intense exercise and don't want to burn out or injure yourself
› You play other sports and/or are extremely active outside of the workouts, and don't want to overtrain

HERE'S WHY YOU MIGHT WANT TO DO THE SUPER ATHLETE PLAN:
› You already consider yourself to be pretty fit; you just want to get even fitter
› These workouts will be your main source of exercise over the next eight weeks
› You want to progress as quickly as possible
› You're willing to put in the hard work in order to see and feel results

Whichever plan you choose, remember: it's all about the intensity. Work hard, be consistent, and continuously challenge yourself, and you'll get fitter, faster, and stronger than ever before.

WARM-UP

Although you may want to skip it if you're in a hurry, warming up before your workout is so important to help you avoid injuries. Warm-ups don't have to be superlong—just long enough to get your muscles moving and your body feeling warmer (hence the term "warm up").

You are welcome to do any pre-workout warm-up exercises you feel like before your workouts, or use the dynamic warm-up outlined here to target every muscle group while getting your heart rate up before crushing your actual workout. In general, your warm-up shouldn't take you more than five to ten minutes to complete, although if you're feeling extra stiff or sore, are coming back from an injury, or the temperature is really cold outside, you might need to spend a little extra time warming up. Learn to listen to your body and adapt to what it needs.

I'm using a band and a jump rope in this warm up, but you can use anything you have around, including a broomstick, PVC pipe, jump rope, etc. If you don't have a jump rope, you can substitute with jumping jacks or just jump in place and pretend you have a rope.

COMPLETE ONE TO TWO ROUNDS, DEPENDING ON HOW WARM YOUR BODY IS FEELING:

- ten wrist rolls each direction
- one hundred single jumps with a jump rope
- five back/front raises
- ten air squats
- two inchworms

WRIST ROLLS

› Clasp your hands together then slowly roll your wrists in a circle.

› Switch directions.

SINGLE-UNDERS

› Complete approximately one hundred single-unders using a jump rope.

› If you don't have a rope, you can pretend to use one while jumping in place, or substitute fifty jumping jacks.

BACK/FRONT RAISES

› Grab a band, jump rope, PVC pipe, or broomstick and grip it about shoulder-width apart or wider, holding it at your thighs.

› Raise your arms up and back until the band is resting at the back of your thighs. The wider your grip, the easier this will be.

AIR SQUATS

› Perform a deep squat, focusing on keeping your core tight, torso upright, and squeezing your glutes on the way up.

INCHWORMS
› From standing, bend down while keeping a slight bend in your knees, then walk your hands forward into a plank position and do a push-up.
› Walk your hands back toward your feet to complete the rep.

COOL-DOWN

Cooling down after a workout helps your body recover faster, and focusing on flexibility exercises, like the ones in this cool-down, will help your body remain mobile and flexible as you build strength.

Ideally, you'll do this cool-down immediately after your workout, but if you're short on time, feel free to do it later in the day—just make sure to do a quick warm-up first so you're not starting completely cold.

I also highly recommend adding foam rolling to your cool-down routine if you're not doing so already.

COMPLETE ONE TO TWO ROUNDS OF THE FOLLOWING STRETCHES

Hold each stretch for thirty to forty-five seconds. Remember to breathe.

RUNNER'S LUNGE STRETCH
If you work out a lot and/or sit a lot during the day, it's almost guaranteed that your hip flexors are tight. This is one of the best stretches for tight hip flexors.
› Get into a lunge position with your forward knee bent over your foot and your back leg extended behind you.
› Tighten your core and squeeze your glutes, and then slowly ease deeper into the stretch, making sure to breathe as you do so.
› You can also reach the arm on your same side up and toward your body to further deepen the stretch.
› Make sure to work both sides.

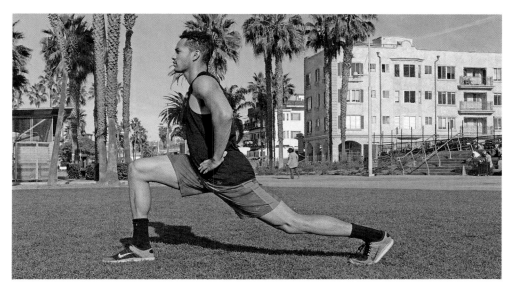

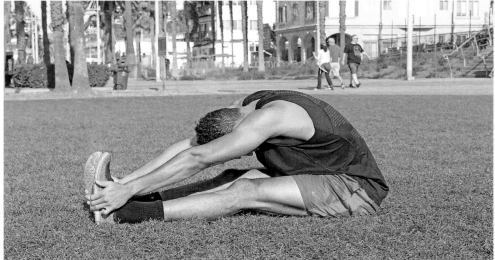

PIKE STRETCH
Beginner Version:

› Sit down with your legs straight in front of you.

› Squeeze your quads, pull your core in, and then fold forward as far as you can.

› Try grabbing the back of your feet for a deeper stretch.

Intermediate Version:

> Stand in front of a wall with your feet together, then lean over and press your upper back against the wall.

> Slowly slide yourself down the wall while keeping your legs as straight as possible.

> The closer you are to the wall, the deeper the stretch will be.

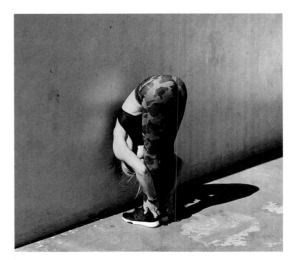

PIGEON STRETCH

This yoga staple is an amazing stretch to open up your hips and really get into your glutes. No matter what your flexibility level or training goal is, you will benefit from this stretch.

> Cross one knee in front of you while keeping the opposite leg straight behind you.

> Place both hands on the ground in front of you and slowly lower your upper body down as much as possible.

> Lower to your forearms if possible.

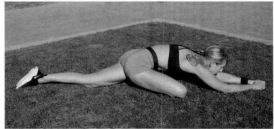

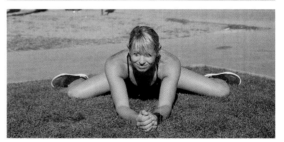

FROG STRETCH

This is a great stretch to help improve flexibility throughout your hips and inner thighs.

> Kneel on the floor with your hands on the ground in front of you.

> Lean forward as you slowly open up your hips into a straddle position, keeping your knees bent as you do so and feet outward in a frog position.

> Lower down as far as you can, leaning your chest toward the floor as you pull your belly button toward your spine. Breathe.

WALL SHOULDER STRETCH

This is one of my absolute favorite stretches to open up the shoulders and chest. Just be prepared: if you're tight in those areas, you will feel it.

> Get in front of a wall and place your hands on the wall above you.

> Slowly lean your chest toward the wall while keeping your hands in place and pulling your core in.

> You should feel like you're trying to get your armpits to touch the wall.

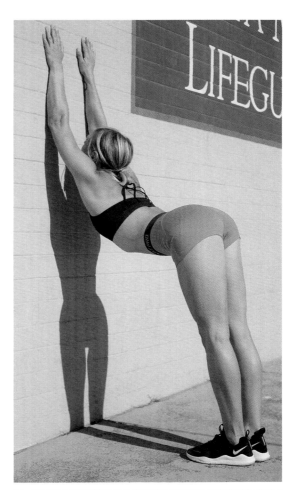

BRIDGE

See pages 126–32 for all bridge variations.

IRON CROSS CHEST AND BACK STRETCH

Most people do a lot of forward and backward movement in their workouts, but very little twisting. This stretch really helps to open up the back and chest at the same time for an incredibly efficient full-body stretch.

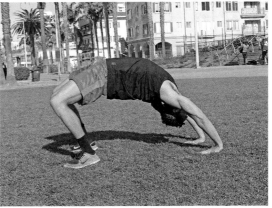

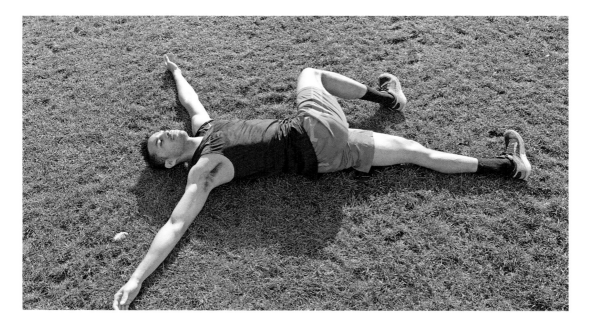

> ‹ Lie on your stomach with one arm stretched to the side.
> ‹ Twist up onto your arm, bringing your top leg behind you.
> ‹ The more you twist, the more you'll open up both your chest and back muscles.
> ‹ Breathe and hold, making sure to stretch both sides.

Note: Avoid this one if you've had disc or lower back injuries in the past.

ADDITIONAL FLEXIBILITY + MOBILITY WORK

Staying flexible and maintaining proper range of motion (ROM) in your body is important not only to be able to do many of the exercises in this book (for example, if you don't have proper shoulder ROM, handstands will be very difficult for you) but also to be able to move better in your daily life. Performing dynamic warm-up exercises before your workout and cooling down afterward with flexibility exercises is one way to address this, and may be enough for some people.

However, if you're excessively tight, have previous injuries, or have other ROM issues, you may need to spend extra time on your flexibility and mobility. This goes beyond the scope of this book, but luckily there are some great resources out there already. Here are some I highly recommend:

› *Becoming a Supple Leopard: The Ultimate Guide to Resolving Pain, Preventing Injury, and Optimizing Athletic Performance*, second edition, Kelly Starrett
› *The Roll Model: A Step-by-Step Guide to Erase Pain, Improve Mobility, and Live Better in Your Body*, Jill Miller
› *The MELT Method: A Breakthrough Self-Treatment System to Eliminate Chronic Pain, Erase the Signs of Aging, and Feel Fantastic in Just 10 Minutes a Day!*, Sue Hitzmann

WORKOUT TYPES

Over the next few pages, you'll see several different types of workouts. Here's what you need to know about them:

TWELVE- AND SIXTEEN-MINUTE WORKOUTS

These workouts take twelve and sixteen minutes, respectively, to complete. You'll need to set an interval timer to the setting for that specific workout. For example, an 18 x :10 x :30 timer setting means you'll set a timer for eighteen rounds of ten-second and thirty-second intervals. You'll rest during the ten-second rest interval, then work as hard as you can during the thirty-second work interval. Go through all rounds until the timer beeps at the end of the workout.

CHALLENGE WORKOUTS

During challenge workouts, you'll go through all the exercises and prescribed number of rounds as fast as possible while maintaining good form. Rest when you need to, but remember, the harder you work, the sooner your workout will be over.

AMRAP WORKOUTS

AMRAP stands for "As Many Rounds As Possible."

You'll need to switch your timer to countdown timer mode, then do as many rounds of the listed exercises as possible within the allotted amount of time. AMRAP workouts are typically no more than twelve minutes, so you have to push as hard as you can in order to get the most out of the workout.

SKILL WORK

Although you can (and will) get stronger and better at the exercises by just doing the HIIT and time challenge workouts in the following pages, if you want to really take your strength and athletic skill set to the next level, you'll need to spend a little extra time building up your skill arsenal. The skill work is optional, so if you don't have an interest or just don't have the time to do the extra work, go ahead and skip it.

Ideally, you'll do your skill work before your workout so that you can give it the proper amount of focus and dedication. But it's also acceptable to do your skill work afterward or at a separate time of the day, as long as you have enough energy not to compromise form.

For example, if the skill work of the day includes handstands, you'll want to work on whichever handstand progression you're currently on with a strong focus on form. If you're working on multiple skills at once, simply go through them as a circuit to save time. For example, your skill workout might look like this:

NUMBER OF ROUNDS: THREE

› 30-second wall handstand hold
› 3 feet-elevated bridge holds

In this example, you would go through each exercise once, then rotate through twice more for a total of three rounds, resting as needed.

> Note: You can choose to follow the Skill Work exactly as prescribed or if you don't have as much time to dedicate to the skill training, you can choose a couple of skills you want to work on now and do the progressions before the regular workouts for the week. If you choose this route, aim to work on each skill work exercise at least twice a week to continue making progress.

EIGHT-WEEK ATHLETE WORKOUT PLAN

ATHLETE WORKOUT PLAN

Example Schedule:

- ✓ Monday—Workout 1
- ✓ Tuesday—Rest
- ✓ Wednesday—Workout 2
- ✓ Thursday—Rest
- ✓ Friday—Workout 3
- ✓ Saturday—Rest
- ✓ Sunday—Rest

✗ Create a plan to best fit your schedule with three workouts a week and rest days in between.

▶▶ WEEK 1

▶▶ *WORKOUT 1*

Skill Work:
Handstands—3 rounds
Bridges—3 rounds

HIIT Workout:
Workout type: 12-minute
Timer setting: 18 x :10 x :30
Equipment: None

Exercises:
Snowboarder jumps
Push-ups
Walking lunges
Burpees
High knees
Rocking planks

▶▶ *WORKOUT 2*

Skill Work:
Push-ups—2 x 15–20 reps
Pull-ups—2 x 8–10 reps
Handstand push-ups—2 x 5 reps

HIIT Workout:
Workout type: 12-minute
Timer setting: 18 x :10 x :30
Equipment: None

Exercises:
Jump lunges
Reptile push-ups
Air squats
High knees
Burpee lateral jumps
V-up in/outs

>> WORKOUT 3

Skill Work:

Pistol squats—3 x 5 reps

Leg raises—3 x 10 reps

Challenge Workout:

Workout type: Challenge

Timer setting: Stopwatch

Equipment: None

Complete three rounds, resting as little as possible in between sets:

10 Long jumps

10 Pike push-ups

20 Walking lunges

10 Burpees

20 Air squats

15 Sit-ups

WEEK 2

>> WORKOUT 1

Skill Work:
Handstands—3 rounds
Bridges—3 rounds

HIIT Workout:
Workout type: 12-minute
Timer setting: 18 x :10 x :30
Equipment: Box

Exercises:
Box jumps
Bulgarian split squats
High knees
Push-ups
Side lunges
Elevated knee touches

>> WORKOUT 2

Skill Work:
Push-ups—2 x 15–20 reps
Pull-ups—2 x 8–10 reps
Handstand push-ups—2 x 5 reps

HIIT Workout:
Workout type: 16-minute
Timer setting: 24 x :10 x :30
Equipment: Jump rope

Exercises:
Single-unders
Boxer push-ups
High knees w/ jump rope
Air squats
Burpees
Rocking planks

➤➤ *WORKOUT 3*

Skill Work:

Pistol squats—3 x 5 reps

Leg raises—3 x 10 reps

Challenge Workout:

Workout type: Challenge

Timer setting: Stopwatch

Equipment: None

Complete four rounds, resting as little as possible in between sets:

1 50-yard sprint (approximately half the length of a football field)

10 Push-ups

20 Walking lunges

30 Pike jumps

10 Candlestick hip bridges / side

10 V-ups

WEEK 3

» WORKOUT 1

Skill Work:

Handstands—3 rounds

Bridges—3 rounds

HIIT Workout:

Workout type: 12-minute

Timer setting: 18 x :10 x :30

Equipment: None

Exercises:

Burpees

Air squats

Pike push-ups

Burpee lateral jumps

Back lunges

V-up in/outs

» WORKOUT 2

Skill Work:

Push-ups—2 x 15–20 reps

Pull-ups—2 x 8–10 reps

Handstand push-ups—2 x 5 reps

HIIT Workout:

Workout type: 16-minute

Timer setting: 24 x :10 x :30

Equipment: Box

Exercises:

Box jumps

Push-ups

Squat step-ups

Burpee box jumps

Mountain climbers

Sit-ups

» *WORKOUT 3*

Skill Work:

Pistol squats—3 x 5 reps

Leg raises—3 x 10 reps

Challenge Workout:

Workout type: Challenge

Timer setting: Stopwatch

Equipment: Parallel bars or equivalent

Complete four rounds, resting as little as possible in between sets:

20 Squat jumps

10 Triceps dips

30 Jump lunges

10 Bodyweight rows

30 Plank hip dips

1 L-sit hold

WEEK 4

>> WORKOUT 1

Skill Work:
Handstands—3 rounds
Bridges—3 rounds

HIIT Workout:
Workout type: 16-minute
Timer setting: 24 x :10 x :30
Equipment: None

Exercises:
Burpees
Push-up hops
Walking lunges
Burpee lateral jumps
Air squats
V-ups

>> WORKOUT 2

Skill Work:
Push-ups—2 x 15–20 reps
Pull-ups—2 x 8–10 reps
Handstand push-ups—2 x 5 reps

HIIT Workout:
Workout type: 12-minute
Timer setting: 18 x :10 x :30
Equipment: Jump rope, box,
    or equivalent

Exercises:
Double-unders *or* single-unders
Side lunges
Crisscross feet w/ jump rope
Step-ups
High knees w/ jump rope
Mountain climbers

» WORKOUT 3

Skill Work:

Pistol squats—3 x 5 reps

Leg raises—3 x 10 reps

Challenge Workout:

Workout type: Challenge

Timer setting: Stopwatch

Equipment: Box, pull-up bar

Complete three rounds, resting as little as possible in between sets:

25 Box jumps

10 Push-ups

5 Pull-ups

20 Air squats

10 Candlestick hip bridges / leg

5 Hanging leg raises

WEEK 5

» WORKOUT 1

Skill Work:
Handstands—3 rounds
Bridges—3 rounds

HIIT Workout:
Workout type: 12-minute
Timer setting: 18 x :10 x :30
Equipment: Jump rope

Exercises:
High knees w/ jump rope
Air squats
Double-unders *or* single-unders
Reptile push-ups
Side-to-side jumps w/ jump rope
Split leg V-ups

» WORKOUT 2

Skill Work:
Push-ups—2 x 15–20 reps
Pull-ups—2 x 8–10 reps
Handstand push-ups—2 x 5 reps

HIIT Workout:
Workout type: 12-minute
Timer setting: 18 x :10 x :30
Equipment: Pull-up bar

Exercises:
Burpee pull-ups
Side lunges
Burpee tuck jumps
Step-ups
Pike push-ups
Twisted hanging knee raises

>> *WORKOUT 3*

Skill Work:
Pistol squats—3 x 5 reps
Leg raises—3 x 10 reps

Challenge Workout:
Workout type: Challenge
Timer setting: Stopwatch
Equipment: None

Complete four rounds, resting as little as possible in between sets:
1 50-yard sprint (approximately half
    the length of a football field)
10 Push-ups
30 Jump lunges
30 Pike jumps
10 Superman raises
10 V-ups

» WEEK 6

» *WORKOUT 1*

Skill Work:
Handstands—3 rounds
Bridges—3 rounds

HIIT Workout:
Workout type: 12-minute
Timer setting: 18 x :10 x :30
Equipment: Box

Exercises:
Box jumps
Decline push-ups
Squat step-ups
Burpee box jumps
Speed step-ups
Elevated knee touches

» *WORKOUT 2*

Skill Work:
Push-ups—2 x 15–20 reps
Pull-ups—2 x 8–10 reps
Handstand push-ups—2 x 5 reps

AMRAP Workout:
Workout type: AMRAP
Timer setting: Countdown from
    12 minutes
Equipment: Jump rope

**Complete as many rounds
as possible in twelve minutes:**
75 High knees w/jump rope
8 Burpees
20 Side lunges
10 Boxer push-ups
20 Air squats
20 V-up in/outs

» *WORKOUT 3*

Skill Work:

Pistol squats—3 x 5 reps

Leg raises—3 x 10 reps

Challenge Workout:

Workout type: Challenge

Timer setting: Stopwatch

Equipment: Pull-up bar, dip bar

Complete three rounds, resting as little as possible in between sets:

5 Burpee pull-ups

10 Squat step-ups

8 Triceps dips

30 Jump lunges

20 Plank hip dips

1 L-sit hold

WEEK 7

» *WORKOUT 1*

Skill Work:

Handstands—3 rounds

Bridges—3 rounds

HIIT Workout:

Workout type: 12-minute

Timer setting: 18 x :10 x :30

Equipment: Jump rope

Exercises:

Double-unders *or* single-unders

Squat jumps

High knees w/ jump rope

Back lunges

Crisscross hands w/ jump rope

V-up in/outs

» *WORKOUT 2*

Skill Work:

Push-ups—2 x 15–20 reps

Pull-ups—2 x 8–10 reps

Handstand push-ups—2 x 5 reps

HIIT Workout:

Workout type: 12-minute

Timer setting: 18 x :10 x :30

Equipment: Box

Exercises:

Sprints *or* high knees

Squat step-ups

Candlestick jump-ups

Pike push-ups

Burpee tuck jumps

Mountain climbers

>> WORKOUT 3

Skill Work:

Pistol squats—3 x 5 reps

Leg raises—3 x 10 reps

Challenge Workout:

Workout type: AMRAP

Timer setting: Countdown from 12
minutes

Equipment: Jump rope

Complete as many rounds as possible in twelve minutes:

50 Double-unders *or* 100 single-
unders

10 Reptile push-ups

20 Walking lunges

100 High knees w/ jump rope

20 Side lunges

10 V-ups

WEEK 8

» WORKOUT 1

Skill Work:

Handstands—3 rounds

Bridges—3 rounds

HIIT Workout:

Workout type: 16-minute

Timer setting: 24 x :10 x :30

Equipment: None

Exercises:

Sprints *or* high knees

Push-up hops

Jump lunges

Burpees

Squat jumps

Split leg V-ups

» WORKOUT 2

Skill Work:

Push-ups—2 x 15–20 reps

Pull-ups—2 x 8–10 reps

Handstand push-ups—2 x 5 reps

AMRAP Workout:

Workout type: AMRAP

Timer setting: Countdown from
    12 minutes

Equipment: Box

**Complete as many rounds
as possible in twelve minutes:**

25 Box jumps

10 Push-up plank jumps

10 Squat step-ups

10 Burpee box jumps

10 V-ups

» *WORKOUT 3*

Skill Work:

Pistol squats—3 x 5 reps

Leg raises—3 x 10 reps

Challenge Workout:

Workout type: Challenge

Timer setting: Stopwatch

Equipment: Pull-up bar, dip bar

Complete three rounds, resting as little as possible in between sets:

5 Pull-ups

20 Squat jumps

10 Triceps dips

20 Side lunges

10 Pike push-ups

10 Hanging leg raises

EIGHT-WEEK SUPER ATHLETE WORKOUT PLAN

SUPER ATHLETE WORKOUT PLAN

Example Schedule:

✓ **Monday—Workout 1**

✓ **Tuesday—Workout 2**

✓ **Wednesday—Workout 3**

✓ **Thursday—Rest**

✓ **Friday—Workout 4**

✓ **Saturday—Workout 5**

✓ **Sunday—Rest**

✗ Create a plan to best fit your schedule with five workouts a week and rest days in between.

WEEK 1

❯❯ WORKOUT 1

Skill Work:
Handstands—3 rounds
Bridges—3 rounds

HIIT Workout:
Workout type: 12-minute
Timer setting: 18 x :10 x :30
Equipment: None

Exercises:
Snowboarder jumps
Push-ups
Walking lunges
Burpees
High knees
Rocking planks

❯❯ WORKOUT 2

Skill Work:
Push-ups—2 x 15–20 reps
Pull-ups—2 x 8–10 reps
Handstand push-ups—2 x 5 reps

HIIT Workout:
Workout type: 12-minute
Timer setting: 18 x :10 x :30
Equipment: None

Exercises:
Jump lunges
Reptile push-ups
Air squats
High knees
Burpee lateral jumps
V-up in/outs

» WORKOUT 3

Skill Work:

Pistol squats—3 x 5 reps

Leg raises—3 x 10 reps

HIIT Workout:

Repeat Workout 1 from this week.

» WORKOUT 4

Skill Work:

Handstands—3 rounds

Bridges—3 rounds

HIIT Workout:

Repeat Workout 2 from this week.

» WORKOUT 5

Skill Work:

Push-ups—2 x 15–20 reps

Pull-ups—2 x 8–10 reps

Handstand push-ups—2 x 5 reps

Challenge Workout:

Workout type: Challenge

Timer setting: Stopwatch

Equipment: None

Repeat three rounds, resting as little as possible in between sets:

10 Long jumps

10 Pike push-ups

20 Walking lunges

10 Burpees

20 Air squats

15 Sit-ups

» WEEK 2

» WORKOUT 1

Skill Work:

Pistol squats—3 x 5 reps

Leg raises—3 x 10 reps

HIIT Workout:

Workout type: 12-minute

Timer setting: 18 x :10 x :30

Equipment: Box

Exercises:

Box jumps

Bulgarian split squats

High knees

Push-ups

Side lunges

Elevated knee touches

» WORKOUT 2

Skill Work:

Handstands—3 rounds

Bridges—3 rounds

HIIT Workout:

Workout type: 16-minute

Timer setting: 24 x :10 x :30

Equipment: Jump rope

Exercises:

Single-unders

Boxer push-ups

High knees w/ jump rope

Air squats

Burpees

Rocking planks

» WORKOUT 3

Skill Work:

Push-ups—2 x 15–20 reps

Pull-ups—2 x 8–10 reps

Handstand push-ups—2 x 5 reps

HIIT Workout:

Repeat Workout 1 from this week.

» WORKOUT 4

Skill Work:

Pistol squats—3 x 5 reps

Leg raises—3 x 10 reps

HIIT Workout:

Repeat Workout 2 from this week.

» WORKOUT 5

Skill Work:

Handstands—3 rounds

Bridges—3 rounds

Challenge Workout:

Workout type: Challenge

Timer setting: Stopwatch

Equipment: None

Complete four rounds, resting as little as possible in between sets:

1 50-yard sprint (approximately half the length of a football field)

10 Push-ups

20 Walking lunges

30 Pike jumps

10 Candlestick hip bridges / side

10 V-ups

WEEK 3

» WORKOUT 1

Skill Work:
Push-ups—2 x 15–20 reps
Pull-ups—2 x 8–10 reps
Handstand push-ups—2 x 5 reps

HIIT Workout:
Workout type: 12-minute
Timer setting: 18 x :10 x :30
Equipment: None

» WORKOUT 2

Skill Work:
Pistol squats—3 x 5 reps
Leg raises—3 x 10 reps

HIIT Workout:
Workout type: 12-minute
Timer setting: 18 x :10 x :30
Equipment: Box

Exercises:
Box jumps
Push-ups
Squat step-ups
Burpee box jumps
Mountain climbers
Sit-ups

» WORKOUT 3

Skill Work:

Handstands—3 rounds

Bridges—3 rounds

HIIT Workout:

Repeat Workout 1 from this week.

» WORKOUT 4

Skill Work:

Push-ups—2 x 15–20 reps

Pull-ups—2 x 8–10 reps

Handstand push-ups—2 x 5 reps

HIIT Workout:

Repeat Workout 2 from this week.

» WORKOUT 5

Skill Work:

Pistol squats—3 x 5 reps

Leg raises—3 x 10 reps

Challenge Workout:

Workout type: Challenge

Timer setting: Stopwatch

Equipment: Parallel bars
  or equivalent

Complete four rounds, resting as little as possible in between sets:

20 Squat jumps

10 Triceps dips

30 Jump lunges

10 Bodyweight rows

30 Plank hip dips

1 L-sit hold

WEEK 4

›› WORKOUT 1

Skill Work:
Handstands—3 rounds
Bridges—3 rounds

HIIT Workout:
Workout type: 16-minute
Timer setting: 24 x :10 x :30
Equipment: None

Exercises:
Burpees
Push-up hops
Walking lunges
Burpee lateral jumps
Air squats
V-ups

›› WORKOUT 2

Skill Work:
Push-ups—2 x 15–20 reps
Pull-ups—2 x 8–10 reps
Handstand push-ups—2 x 5 reps

HIIT Workout:
Workout type: 12-minute
Timer setting: 18 x :10 x :30
Equipment: Jump rope, box,
  or equivalent

Exercises:
Double-unders *or* single-unders
Side lunges
Crisscross feet w/ jump rope
Step-ups
High knees w/ jump rope
Mountain climbers

>> WORKOUT 3

Skill Work:

Pistol squats—3 x 5 reps

Leg raises—3 x 10 reps

HIIT Workout:

Repeat Workout 1 from this week.

>> WORKOUT 4

Skill Work:

Handstands—3 rounds

Bridges—3 rounds

HIIT Workout:

Repeat Workout 2 from this week.

>> WORKOUT 5

Skill Work:

Push-ups—2 x 15–20 reps

Pull-ups—2 x 8–10 reps

Handstand push-ups—2 x 5 reps

Challenge Workout:

Workout type: Challenge

Timer setting: Stopwatch

Equipment: Box, pull-up bar

Complete three rounds, resting as little as possible in between sets:

25 Box jumps

10 Push-ups

5 Pull-ups

20 Air squats

10 Candlestick hip bridges / leg

5 Hanging leg raises

» WEEK 5

» WORKOUT 1

Skill Work:

Pistol squats—3 x 5 reps

Leg raises—3 x 10 reps

HIIT Workout:

Workout type: 12-minute

Timer setting: 18 x :10 x :30

Equipment: Jump rope

Exercises:

High knees w/ jump rope

Air squats

Double-unders *or* single-unders

Reptile push-ups

Side to side jumps w/ jump rope

Split leg V-ups

» WORKOUT 2

Skill Work:

Handstands—3 rounds

Bridges—3 rounds

HIIT Workout:

Workout type: 12-minute

Timer setting: 18 x :10 x :30

Equipment: Pull-up bar

Exercises:

Burpee pull-ups

Side lunges

Burpee tuck jumps

Step-ups

Pike push-ups

Twisted hanging knee raises

❯❯ *WORKOUT 3*

Skill Work:

Push-ups—2 x 15–20 reps
Pull-ups—2 x 8–10 reps
Handstand push-ups—2 x 5 reps

HIIT Workout:

Repeat Workout 1 from this week.

❯❯ *WORKOUT 4*

Skill Work:

Pistol squats—3 x 5 reps
Leg raises—3 x 10 reps

HIIT Workout:

Repeat Workout 2 from this week.

❯❯ *WORKOUT 5*

Skill Work:

Handstands—3 rounds
Bridges—3 rounds

Challenge Workout:

Workout type: Challenge
Timer setting: Stopwatch
Equipment: None

Complete four rounds, resting as little as possible in between sets:

1 50-yard sprint (approximately half the length of a football field)
10 Push-ups
30 Jump lunges
30 Pike jumps
10 Superman raises
10 V-ups

» WEEK 6

» WORKOUT 1

Skill Work:
Push-ups—2 x 15–20 reps
Pull-ups—2 x 8–10 reps
Handstand push-ups—2 x 5 reps

HIIT Workout:
Workout type: 12-minute
Timer setting: 18 x :10 x :30
Equipment: Box

Exercises:
Box jumps
Decline push-ups
Squat step-ups
Burpee box jumps
Speed step-ups
Elevated knee touches

» WORKOUT 2

Skill Work:
Pistol squats—3 x 5 reps
Leg raises—3 x 10 reps

AMRAP Workout:
Workout type: AMRAP
Timer setting: Count down from
        12 minutes
Equipment: Jump rope

Complete as many rounds as possible in twelve minutes:
75 high knees w/ jump rope
8 burpees
20 side lunges
10 boxer push-ups
20 air squats
20 V-up in/outs

» WORKOUT 3

Skill Work:

Handstands—3 rounds

Bridges—3 rounds

HIIT Workout:

Repeat Workout 1 from this week.

» WORKOUT 4

Skill Work:

Push-ups—2 x 15–20 reps

Pull-ups—2 x 8–10 reps

Handstand push-ups—2 x 5 reps

AMRAP Workout:

Repeat Workout 2 from this week.

» WORKOUT 5

Skill Work:

Pistol squats—3 x 5 reps

Leg raises—3 x 10 reps

Challenge Workout:

Workout type: Challenge

Timer setting: Stopwatch

Equipment: Pull-up bar, box,
   dip bar

Complete three rounds, resting as little as possible in between sets:

5 Burpee pull-ups

10 Squat step ups

8 Triceps dips

30 Jump lunges

20 Plank hip dips

1 L-sit hold

WEEK 7

» WORKOUT 1

Skill Work:
Handstands—3 rounds
Bridges—3 rounds

HIIT Workout:
Workout type: 12-minute
Timer setting: 18 x :10 x :30
Equipment: Jump rope

Exercises:
Double-unders *or* single-unders
Squat jumps
High knees w/ jump rope
Back lunges
Crisscross hands w/ jump rope
V-up in/outs

» WORKOUT 2

Skill Work:
Push-ups—2 x 15–20 reps
Pull-ups—2 x 8–10 reps
Handstand push-ups—2 x 5 reps

HIIT Workout:
Workout type: 12-minute
Timer setting: 18 x :10 x :30
Equipment: Box

Exercises:
Sprints *or* high knees
Squat step-ups
Candlestick jump-ups
Pike push-ups
Burpee tuck jumps
Mountain climbers

» WORKOUT 3

Skill Work:

Pistol squats—3 x 5 reps

Leg raises—3 x 10 reps

HIIT Workout:

Repeat Workout 1 from this week.

» WORKOUT 4

Skill Work:

Handstands—3 rounds

Bridges—3 rounds

HIIT Workout:

Repeat Workout 2 from this week.

» WORKOUT 5

Skill Work:

Push-ups—2 x 15–20 reps

Pull-ups—2 x 8–10 reps

Handstand push-ups—2 x 5 reps

AMRAP Workout:

Workout type: AMRAP

Timer setting: Count down from
    12 minutes

Equipment: Jump rope

**Complete as many rounds
as possible in twelve minutes:**

50 Double-unders *or*
    100 single-unders

10 Reptile push-ups

20 Walking lunges

100 High knees w/ jump rope

20 Side lunges

10 V-ups

WEEK 8

>> WORKOUT 1

Skill Work:

Pistol squats—3 x 5 reps

Leg raises—3 x 10 reps

HIIT Workout:

Workout type: 16-minute

Timer setting: 24 x :10 x :30

Equipment: None

Exercises:

Sprints *or* high knees

Push-up hops

Jump lunges

Burpees

Squat jumps

Split-leg V-ups

>> WORKOUT 2

Skill Work:

Handstands—3 rounds

Bridges—3 rounds

AMRAP Workout:

Workout type: AMRAP

Timer setting: Count down from
    12 minutes

Equipment: Box

Complete as many rounds as possible in twelve minutes:

25 box jumps

10 push-up plank jumps

10 squat step-ups

10 burpee box jumps

10 v-ups

» WORKOUT 3

Skill Work:

Push-ups—2 x 15–20 reps

Pull-ups—2 x 8–10 reps

Handstand push-ups—2 x 5 reps

HIIT Workout:

Repeat Workout 1 from this week.

» WORKOUT 4

Skill Work:

Pistol squats—3 x 5 reps

Leg raises—3 x 10 reps

AMRAP Workout:

Repeat Workout 2 from this week.

» WORKOUT 5

Skill Work:

Handstands—3 rounds

Bridges—3 rounds

Challenge Workout:

Workout type: Challenge

Timer setting: Stopwatch

Equipment: Pull-up bar, dip bar

Complete three rounds, resting as little as possible in between sets:

5 Pull-ups

20 Squat jumps

10 Triceps dips

20 Side lunges

10 Pike push-ups

10 Hanging leg raises

BONUS: TABATA WORKOUTS

Whether you just want an extra finisher to top off your regular workout, or you *actually* don't have twelve minutes to spare for a full HIIT workout, Tabata workouts are an extremely efficient way to get a workout in—and they only take four minutes to complete.

Developed by Dr. Izumi Tabata at the National Institute of Fitness and Sports in Tokyo, Japan, Tabata training can increase your overall aerobic and anaerobic capacity, VO_2 max, resting metabolic rate, and help you burn more fat—in just four minutes flat.

The only caveat? During Tabata training you have to work really, really hard during the entire four minutes.

To do a Tabata workout, you'll set an interval timer to eight rounds of 10-second and 20-second intervals. You'll be resting on the 10-second intervals, then working as hard as you possibly can on the 20-second ones.

Here are eight incredibly efficient, fat-blasting, heart-pumping Tabata workouts you can do nearly anywhere.

#1: SPRINT TABATA

Tabata Workout:

Timer setting: 8 x :10 x :20

Equipment: None

This is the classic Tabata workout, and the one most people think of when they think of Tabatas. To do it, just find an open space and set your timer for eight rounds of ten and twenty seconds.

Then sprint your heart out during the twenty-second intervals and walk or rest completely during the ten-second intervals.

#2: JUMP ROPE TABATA

Tabata Workout:

Timer setting: 8 x :10 x :20

Equipment: Jump rope

Another awesome cardio Tabata, this is my go-to Tabata workout when I want to make sure I have nothing left to give after a workout.

To do it, set your timer for eight rounds of ten and twenty seconds, then perform high knees with a jump rope as fast as you possibly can during the twenty-second intervals and rest during the ten-second intervals.

#3: ALTERNATE BETWEEN: BURPEES + MOUNTAIN CLIMBERS

Tabata Workout:

Timer setting: 8 x :10 x :20

Equipment: None

This Tabata workout adds an extra challenge: you'll be doing two different exercises and switching every other interval.

You'll start by doing twenty seconds of burpees, rest, and then do twenty seconds of mountain climbers. Continue until you've completed all eight rounds.

#4: ALTERNATE BETWEEN: SQUAT JUMPS + PIKE JUMPS

Tabata Workout:

Timer setting: 8 x :10 x :20

Equipment: None

Start with twenty seconds of squat jumps, rest, and then do twenty seconds of pike jumps. Continue until you've completed all eight rounds.

#5: ALTERNATE BETWEEN: AIR SQUATS + PUSH-UPS

Tabata Workout:

Timer setting: 8 x :10 x :20

Equipment: None

Start with twenty seconds of air squats, rest, and then do twenty seconds of push-ups. Continue until you've completed all eight rounds.

#6: ALTERNATE BETWEEN: SNOWBOARDER JUMPS + PLANK JUMPS

Tabata Workout:

Timer setting: 8 x :10 x :20

Equipment: None

Start with twenty seconds of snowboarder jumps, rest, and then do twenty seconds of plank jumps. Continue switching back and forth for the entire four minutes.

#7: ALTERNATE BETWEEN: AIR SQUATS + PUSH-UPS

Tabata Workout:

Timer setting: 8 x :10 x :20

Equipment: None

Start with twenty seconds of air squats, rest, and then do twenty seconds of push-ups. Continue until you've completed all eight rounds.

#8: ALTERNATE BETWEEN: HIGH KNEES + MOUNTAIN CLIMBERS (NO REST)

Tabata Workout:

Timer setting: 8 x :10 x :20

Equipment: None

This one will leave you breathless and wondering how four minutes could possibly take so long.

Start with twenty seconds of high knees. Then, instead of resting during the ten seconds, drop down and do mountain climbers instead. Repeat. Continue for the entire four minutes, taking no rest.

RECIPES

EASY HEALTHY BREAKFASTS

**QUICK & HEALTHY
SNACKS & SMOOTHIES**

HEALTHY TREATS

APPLE BANANA CHIA SEED MUFFINS

Nutrition Facts (per muffin)

Calories: 113   Total carbohydrates: 17.5g

Total fat: 2.5g   Protein: 6.5g

Ingredients:

1 cup old-fashioned oats

½ cup vanilla whey protein powder

½ cup unsweetened almond, oat, or regular milk

2 tbsp cottage cheese**

2 tbsp chia seeds

1 tsp vanilla extract

1 tsp cinnamon

1 tsp baking powder

¼ tsp salt

1 large ripe banana

1 egg*

2–3 dates, pitted

1 medium apple, peeled and diced

Directions:

1. Heat your oven to 350° Fahrenheit. While the oven is warming, blend everything together except for the apple, using a blender or hand mixer until there are no remaining chunks.

2. Stir the apple into the batter, then pour the mixture into eight silicone baking cups.

3. Put into the oven and bake for about 20 to 22 minutes, or until the muffins are slightly browned on top.

4. Eat warmed or chilled, and slather with nut butter, Greek yogurt, or your favorite topping.

5. Store any leftover muffins in the refrigerator or freezer.

Note on protein powders: Depending on the type of protein powder you're using, you may need to adjust the amount of liquid added since different protein powders soak up liquids differently. If the recipe seems too dry, add additional liquid in a teaspoon at a time until you can mix everything together. If it seems too liquidy, add additional flour or oats until you reach the desired thickness.

In my experience, vegan blend protein powders work better than single-source vegan powders for baking.

If you'd prefer to omit protein powders altogether, simply replace with additional flour or oats

*VEGAN: Replace eggs with flax eggs. 1 flax egg = 1 tbs ground flax + 3 tbsp water

**VEGAN: Replace cottage cheese or Greek yogurt in recipes with mashed ripe banana

FOUR-INGREDIENT PROTEIN PANCAKES

Nutrition Facts (per entire recipe)
Calories: 350   Total carbohydrates: 34g

Total fat: 6g   Protein: 36g

Ingredients:

½ cup old fashioned oats

½ cup cottage cheese**

¾ cup egg whites*

1 tsp vanilla extract

Directions:

1. Using a hand mixer or blender, blend all of the ingredients together so that there are no remaining chunks of oatmeal or cottage cheese.

2. Heat a nonstick pan over medium-high heat, then pour the batter into your desired pancake shapes once the pan is hot. Keep in mind that smaller pancakes are much easier to flip.

3. As soon as small bubbles start forming on the pancakes and they're lightly browned on one side, use a spatula to flip the pancakes.

4. Fully cook the other side, then add your favorite toppings.

EASY HEALTHY BREAKFASTS

BANANA-BLUEBERRY FLAX PROTEIN PANCAKES

Nutrition Facts (per recipe)

Calories: 350	Total carbohydrates: 60g
Total fat: 6g	Protein: 18g

Ingredients:

1 large ripe banana

1 tsp vanilla extract

½ cup pea protein milk or milk of your choice

½ cup oat flour (make your own by blending regular oats in a blender)

¼ cup egg whites*

1 tbsp flax seeds, ground

¼ tsp baking powder

½ tsp cinnamon

¼ tsp sea salt

¼ cup blueberries, fresh or frozen

Directions:

1. Whisk together the banana, vanilla extract, and pea protein milk.

2. Add in the oat flour, egg whites, flax seeds, baking powder, cinnamon, and sea salt.

3. Stir the mixture until there are no remaining banana chunks.

4. Heat a lightly greased pan over medium-low heat, then pour the mixture onto the pan in desired pancake shapes.

5. Wait about a minute, then sprinkle a spoonful of blueberries on top of each pancake, using the back of the spoon to gently press the blueberries down into the pancakes.

6. Once the edges are firm and the middle begins to bubble, flip the pancake.

7. Let cook for a couple of minutes, then transfer to a plate.

8. Continue this until all the batter is used up.

9. Top with more blueberries, maple syrup, or your favorite pancake toppings.

*VEGAN: Replace eggs with flax eggs. 1 flax egg = 1 tbs ground flax + 3 tbsp water
**VEGAN: Replace cottage cheese or Greek yogurt in recipes with mashed ripe banana

YEAR-ROUND PUMPKIN PROTEIN PANCAKES

Nutrition Facts (per entire recipe)

Calories: 380   Total carbohydrates: 42g

Total fat: 7.5g   Protein: 33.5g

Ingredients:

½ cup egg whites*

½ cup old fashioned oats

½ cup pumpkin puree

¼ cup almond, oat, or other milk of your choice

¼ cup whey protein powder

1 tbsp ground flax seeds

1 tsp vanilla extract

1 tsp baking soda

1 tsp pumpkin pie spice

Directions:

1. Using a hand mixer or blender, blend all of the ingredients together until you have a smooth batter.

2. Heat a nonstick pan over medium-high heat, then pour the batter into your desired pancake shapes once the pan is hot. Keep in mind that smaller pancakes are much easier to flip.

3. As soon as small bubbles start forming on the pancakes and they're lightly browned on one side, use a spatula to flip the pancakes.

4. Fully cook the other side, then add your favorite toppings.

EASY HEALTHY BREAKFASTS

LEMON–CHIA SEED PROTEIN MUFFINS

Nutrition Facts (per muffin)

Calories: 115   Total carbohydrates: 18g

Total fat: 2g   Protein: 7g

Ingredients:

Juice and zest of one small Meyer lemon

½ tsp baking powder

1 cup oat flour (make your own by blending regular oats in a blender)

½ cup vanilla whey protein powder

½ cup unsweetened applesauce

¼ cup Greek yogurt**

¼ cup honey or maple syrup

1 egg*

1 tbsp chia seeds

½ tsp salt

Directions:

1. Heat your oven to 350° Fahrenheit.

2. While the oven is heating up, put the lemon juice and zest in a small bowl, and add the baking powder and mix.

3. In a separate medium-sized bowl, stir together the oat flour, protein powder, applesauce, Greek yogurt, honey, egg, chia seeds, and salt.

4. Add the lemon mixture to the medium bowl and stir well.

5. Pour into eight silicone baking cups and bake for about 20 minutes or until slightly browned on top.

*VEGAN: Replace eggs with flax eggs. 1 flax egg = 1 tbs ground flax + 3 tbsp water
**VEGAN: Replace cottage cheese or Greek yogurt in recipes with mashed ripe banana

HEARTY OATMEAL-APPLESAUCE PROTEIN PANCAKES

Nutrition Facts (per entire recipe)

Calories: 320   Total carbohydrates: 27g

Total fat: 3.5g   Protein: 44g

Ingredients:

1 serving whey or vegan blend protein powder

½ cup old-fashioned oats

⅓ cup unsweetened applesauce

2 egg whites*

¼ cup cottage cheese**

1 tsp vanilla extract

½ tsp cinnamon

¼ tsp baking powder

Directions:

1. Using a hand mixer or blender, blend all of the ingredients together until there are no remaining chunks of oatmeal or cottage cheese.

2. Heat a nonstick pan over medium-high heat, then pour the batter into your desired pancake shapes once the pan is hot. Keep in mind that smaller pancakes are much easier to flip.

3. As soon as small bubbles start forming on the pancakes and they're lightly browned on one side, use a spatula to flip the pancakes.

4. Fully cook the other side, then add your favorite toppings.

EASY HEALTHY BREAKFASTS

MORNING CHOCOLATE CHIP BANANA OAT MUFFINS

Nutrition Facts (per muffin)

Calories: 115   Total carbohydrates: 18g

Total fat: 2.5g   Protein: 6g

Ingredients:

1 cup old-fashioned oats

1 large ripe banana

½ cup vanilla whey or pea protein powder

1 egg*

¼ cup milk or milk substitute

2 tbsp cottage cheese**

1 tsp vanilla extract

½ tsp cinnamon

½ tsp baking powder

¼ tsp salt

2–3 dates, pitted

2 tbsp mini chocolate chips

Directions:

1. Heat your oven to 350° Fahrenheit.

2. Using a hand mixer or blender, blend together all of the ingredients except for the chocolate chips until there are no remaining chunks.

3. Stir in the chocolate chips, then pour into eight silicone baking cups.

4. Bake for about 35 minutes or until slightly browned on top. Enjoy at room temperature or warmed with your favorite nut butter spread on top.

5. Store any leftover muffins in the refrigerator or freezer.

*VEGAN: Replace eggs with flax eggs. 1 flax egg = 1 tbs ground flax + 3 tbsp water
**VEGAN: Replace cottage cheese or Greek yogurt in recipes with mashed ripe banana

PUMPKIN–CHOCOLATE CHIP PROTEIN MUFFINS

Nutrition Facts (per muffin)

Calories: 115   Total carbohydrates: 18g

Total fat: 2g   Protein: 7g

Ingredients:

1 cup old fashioned oats

¾ cup pumpkin puree (not pumpkin pie mix)

1 serving vanilla whey protein powder

⅓ cup honey or maple syrup

¼ cup almond, oat, or regular milk

2 tbsp cottage cheese**

1 tsp vanilla extract

½ tsp cinnamon

½ tsp pumpkin pie spice

½ tsp baking powder

½ tsp salt

1 egg*

¼ cup mini dark chocolate chips

Directions:

1. Heat your oven to 325° Fahrenheit.

2. While the oven is heating up, use a mixer or hand blender to blend together all of the ingredients except for the chocolate chips in a medium-sized bowl until there are no remaining chunks.

3. Stir in the chocolate chips evenly throughout the mixture.

4. Pour into eight silicone or regular muffin liners, filling to the brim.

5. Put into the oven and bake for about 40 minutes, or until they get slightly browned on top. Note that they'll still be a little gooey when you take them out. Let them cool, then stick in the refrigerator to chill.

6. Store any remaining muffins in the refrigerator or freezer.

EASY HEALTHY BREAKFASTS

APPLE CINNAMON ENERGY BALLS

Nutrition Facts (per ⅛ recipe)

Calories: 140   Total carbohydrates: 16.5g

Total fat: 5.5g   Protein: 7g

Ingredients:

¼ cup unsweetened almond butter

2 tbsp honey or maple syrup

1 cup old-fashioned oats

1 scoop vanilla whey protein powder

1½ tsp cinnamon

½ tsp nutmeg

1 small apple, finely diced

Directions:

1. In a medium-sized bowl, stir together the almond butter and honey.

2. Add in the oats, protein powder, cinnamon, and nutmeg, and stir until all ingredients are evenly distributed.

3. Next, stir in the diced apple.

4. If the mixture isn't sticking together quite right, just add a little more almond butter or honey until it's sticky enough that you can mold it into eight small 1- to 2-inch balls. If it seems too moist, add additional oats one tablespoon at a time until you get a workable dough.

5. Place the bites on parchment paper and stick them in the refrigerator for one to two hours or until chilled.

CASHEW CHERRY CHUNK ENERGY BARS

Nutrition Facts (per ¼ recipe)

Calories: 170   Total carbohydrates: 18g

Total fat: 8.5g   Protein: 5g

Ingredients:

½ cup crisp rice or millet cereal

¼ cup quick-cooking rolled oats

¼ cup vanilla whey protein powder

1 tsp cinnamon

Pinch of sea salt

2 tbsp almond butter

1 tbsp honey or maple syrup

2 tbsp unsweetened almond milk

2 tbsp cashews, coarsely chopped

2 tbsp unsweetened dried cherries, coarsely chopped

2 tbsp dark chocolate chips or chopped chocolate bar

Coconut oil, for greasing parchment paper

Directions:

1. Stir the rice cereal, oats, protein powder, cinnamon, and sea salt together in a medium-sized bowl.

2. Add in the almond butter, honey, and almond milk and mix thoroughly.

3. Next, stir in the cashews, cherries, and chocolate chips until everything is incorporated evenly.

4. Lightly spread a little coconut oil on parchment paper and place the dough on top.

5. Use the parchment paper to flatten the dough so that it's in a fairly rectangular shape—remember, this will be the eventual thickness of your bars.

6. Place the dough in the refrigerator for an hour or so, then cut into four evenly sized bars.

7. Wrap in foil and store bars in the fridge or freezer.

QUICK AND HEALTHY SNACKS AND SMOOTHIES

CHOCOLATE-DRIZZLED PISTACHIO PROTEIN BARS

Nutrition Facts (per ¼ recipe)

Calories: 230   Total carbohydrates: 20g

Total fat: 15g   Protein: 9g

Ingredients:

¼ cup almond butter

1 tbsp honey or maple syrup

3–4 tbsp unsweetened almond milk

¾ cup millet puffs or puffed rice cereal

½ cup old-fashioned oats

¼ cup vanilla whey protein powder

2 tbsp pistachios, chopped

Coconut oil, for greasing the wax paper

4 squares high-quality dark chocolate

Pinch of sea salt

Directions:

1. Mix the almond butter, honey, and almond milk in a medium-sized bowl.

2. Add in the millet puffs, oats, and protein powder and mix well.

3. Stir in about two-thirds of the chopped pistachios until they're evenly spread throughout the mixture.

4. Next, lightly coat a sheet of wax paper with coconut oil and form four bars. You can chill the dough slightly beforehand if you want to make it easier to work with; otherwise just fold the wax paper over the bars to help flatten them.

5. Melt the chocolate in the microwave or on the stovetop, then drizzle equally over each bar.

6. Immediately sprinkle on the remaining pistachios and sea salt and use your fingers to lightly press onto the tops of the bars.

7. Place in the fridge and chill for at least an hour.

8. Wrap in foil and store bars in the fridge or freezer.

HEALTHY HIGH-PROTEIN MOCHA FREEZE

Nutrition Facts (per entire recipe)

Calories: 220   Total carbohydrates: 23g

Total fat: 3.5g   Protein: 28g

Ingredients:

1 serving chocolate protein powder

½ cup almond, oat, or regular milk

1–2 tbsp unsweetened cocoa powder

2 ounces cold brewed coffee or two shots of espresso

Handful of ice cubes

Directions:

1. Add the protein powder, milk of your choice, cocoa powder, coffee, and ice, and blend thoroughly.

2. If the drink seems too runny, add more ice; and if it seems too chunky, add more milk.

QUICK AND HEALTHY SNACKS AND SMOOTHIES

PB&J SMOOTHIE

Nutrition Facts (per entire recipe)

Calories: 370   Total carbohydrates: 42g

Total fat: 12g   Protein: 29g

Ingredients:

1 serving whey or vegan protein powder

1 small frozen banana

½ cup frozen strawberries

½ cup unsweetened coconut milk
in a carton

1 tbsp chunky or natural peanut butter

Handful of ice

Directions:

1. Blend all the ingredients together and serve chilled. Add more ice if too runny; more coconut milk if too thick.

PIÑA COLADA SMOOTHIE

Nutrition Facts (per entire recipe)

Calories: 330   Total carbohydrates: 21g

Total fat: 10g   Protein: 25.5g

Ingredients:

1 serving whey or vegan protein powder

½ cup frozen pineapple

1 cup unsweetened coconut milk
in a carton

½ frozen banana

1 tsp coconut butter

Handful of ice cubes

Directions:

1. Blend all the ingredients together and serve chilled. Add more ice if too runny; more coconut milk if too thick.

QUICK AND HEALTHY
SNACKS AND SMOOTHIES

SEVEN-INGREDIENT OATMEAL PEANUT BUTTER ENERGY BARS

Nutrition Facts (per ¼ recipe)

Calories: 230   Total carbohydrates: 18g

Total fat: 11.5g   Protein: 14.5g

Ingredients:

¼ cup almond, oat, or regular milk

¼ cup natural chunky peanut butter

1 tsp vanilla extract

1 cup old-fashioned oats

⅔ cup vanilla whey protein powder

½ tsp cinnamon

2 tbsp dark chocolate chips

Coconut oil, for greasing the parchment paper

Directions:

1. Stir the almond milk, peanut butter, and vanilla in a medium-sized bowl.

2. Add in the oats, protein powder, and cinnamon and stir until there are no remaining chunks.

3. Add in the chocolate chips, mixing evenly throughout the dough.

4. If the mixture seems too dry, add in a little more milk, one tablespoon at a time.

5. If the mixture seems too gooey, add in a few extra oats, one tablespoon at a time.

6. Line a 4×8-inch pan with parchment paper, spray with a little coconut oil, then spread the dough so that it's pressed down evenly into the pan.

7. Use your hands or a spatula to flatten the top of the dough.

8. Place the mixture in the fridge for one to two hours or until chilled.

9. Once the bars are chilled, cut them into four pieces, and wrap each individually in foil or plastic wrap.

10. Store any remaining bars in the fridge or freezer.

CHOCOLATE-COVERED PEANUT BUTTER PROTEIN BALLS

Nutrition Facts (per $\frac{1}{12}$ recipe)

Calories: 100   Total carbohydrates: 4g

Total fat: 6.5g   Protein: 6.5g

Ingredients:

2 servings whey protein powder

6 tbsp chunky natural peanut butter

3–4 tbsp almond milk
or milk of your choice

Approximately 60 grams high-quality
dark chocolate

Directions:

1. Add the protein powder and peanut butter to a medium-sized bowl (if you want to make the stirring a little easier, melt the peanut butter in the microwave for 10 to 15 seconds beforehand).

2. Stir in two tablespoons of almond milk, and add an additional one or two tablespoons until everything is mixed together well and there are no remaining dry chunks. Don't add too much liquid— the mixture should be very sticky, but not runny at all.

3. Form twelve 1- to 2-inch balls out of the mixture and place them on wax paper to keep them from sticking. Cover and put in the refrigerator for at least 30 minutes.

4. Once the peanut butter balls are chilled, remove them from the refrigerator and melt the chocolate over a stovetop or using a microwave, being careful not to burn the chocolate.

5. While the chocolate is still melted, dip the peanut butter balls in the chocolate, covering them completely. Return to the wax paper, cover, and place in the refrigerator.

HEALTHY TREATS

EASY DARK CHOCOLATE ALMOND BUTTER CUPS

Nutrition Facts (per 1/10 recipe)

Calories: 130   Total carbohydrates: 6g

Total fat: 10.5g   Protein: 3g

Ingredients:

½ cup smooth almond butter

1 tbsp honey, warmed

1 tbsp coconut oil, melted

40 grams high-quality dark chocolate

Pinch of sea salt

Directions:

1. Use a hand blender or food processor to blend together the almond butter, honey, and coconut oil until you get a smooth paste.

2. Melt the chocolate, then pour half into ten silicone baking cups and put into the freezer for 5 to 10 minutes or until chocolate is set.

3. Evenly spoon the almond butter mixture into the cups, using your fingers or a spoon to make each one level (it helps to wet your fingers first).

4. Next, pour the remaining chocolate into each cup, picking up and swirling it around until the chocolate covers all the almond butter mixture.

5. Immediately sprinkle sea salt on top and place in the freezer for 30 minutes or until firm.

6. Store in the fridge or freezer (if you have any leftovers!).

VANILLA PISTACHIO PROTEIN TRUFFLES

Nutrition Facts (per ¹⁄₁₀ recipe)

Calories: 100   Total carbohydrates: 15g

Total fat: 4g   Protein: 6g

Ingredients:

⅔ cup oat flour (or just blend some oats to make your own)

½ cup vanilla whey protein powder

¼ cup unsweetened almond, oat, or regular milk

2 tbsp coconut flour

2 tbsp maple syrup or honey

½ tsp vanilla extract

60 grams (about ¼ bar) high-quality dark chocolate

5 pistachios (or ½ tbsp), finely chopped

Directions:

1. Combine the oat flour, protein powder, milk, coconut flour, maple syrup, and vanilla extract in a bowl.

2. Mix everything together until there are no remaining chunks, then form into ten round balls using your hands to roll them together. Place on wax paper, then chill in the refrigerator for at least 30 to 60 minutes.

3. While the dough is chilling, melt the chocolate in the microwave or on the stovetop, being careful not to burn it.

4. Remove the dough from the fridge, then one at a time, coat the truffles in chocolate, then generously sprinkle with pistachios, using your fingers to press the pistachio pieces into the chocolate.

5. Place back in the fridge to chill, then eat up!

HEALTHY TREATS

THE EASIEST (HEALTHY) 5-INGREDIENT COOKIE EVER

Nutrition Facts (per ¹/₁₀ recipe)

Calories: 52   Total carbohydrates: 9.5g

Total fat: 1g   Protein: 1g

Ingredients:

1 large ripe banana

1 cup old-fashioned oats

1 tsp cinnamon

2 tbsp chocolate chips, dried cherries, or other dried fruit

1 tbsp walnuts, chopped (optional)

Directions:

1. Heat your oven to 350° Fahrenheit.

2. While the oven is heating up, mash the banana and oats together so that there are no chunks of banana left and every single oat is covered (since this recipe doesn't use any liquid, you'll want to pay special attention to this since you don't want to bite into any dry oats once they're done baking).

3. Next, stir in the cinnamon, chocolate chips, and walnuts. Take an ice cream scoop or a large spoon and mold ten miniature cookie balls onto a lightly greased cookie sheet or a cooking mat.

4. Place in the oven and let bake for about 20 minutes, or until they're slightly browned on the bottom.

5. Serve while warm.

SUPER EASY BERRY CRUMBLE

Nutrition Facts (per ½ recipe)

Calories: 270   Total carbohydrates: 43g

Total fat: 9g   Protein: 6g

Ingredients:

1½ cups fresh or frozen berries such as blueberries, raspberries, blackberries, or marionberries (or a mixture)

½ tsp cornstarch, potato starch, or tapioca starch for thickening

⅓ cup old-fashioned oats

2 tbsp coconut sugar

2 tbsp whole wheat flour or oat flour

1 tsp cinnamon

Pinch of sea salt

2 tbsp almond, oat, or regular milk

1 tbsp coconut oil, melted

Directions:

1. Heat your oven to 350° Fahrenheit.

2. Mix the berries and cornstarch together in a medium-sized bowl.

3. In a separate bowl, mix together the oats, coconut sugar, whole-wheat flour, cinnamon, and salt.

4. Stir in the almond milk and coconut oil until it forms a crumbly mixture.

5. Pour the berry mixture evenly into single-serving ceramic ramekins, then sprinkle the oat mixture on top of each and place into the oven.

6. Bake for about 25 to 30 minutes or until the tops are slightly browned and the berries start to bubble on the sides.

7. Let sit to cool slightly, then serve while still warm. Top with a scoop of ice cream or frozen yogurt for an extra treat!

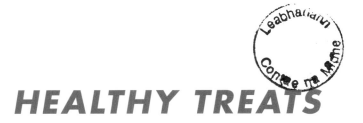

HEALTHY TREATS

ACKNOWLEDGMENTS

Thank you, from the bottom of my heart, to all the amazing people in my life.

Brian, thank you for encouraging me and believing in me no matter what. My parents, thank you for instilling in me the love of lifelong learning, giving me the travel bug, and for letting me take my own path, even when it wasn't easy. My big brother, for always messing with me and not letting me grow up to be a total wimp. My big sister, for showing me at a young age that women could be smart and capable, and for always making me laugh.

Amy Mitchell, thank you for all of your encouragement and for always pushing me to get out of my comfort zone.

My furry kids, Rocket and Fishstick, thank you for keeping me company and never, ever failing to make me smile.

Thank you to all of my teachers growing up for encouraging me to write.

Thank you to all of the trainers and coaches I've worked with along my own fitness journey for showing me what's possible.

Thank you to the 12 Minute Athlete community, especially those of you who have been there from the very beginning. You all ROCK.

INDEX

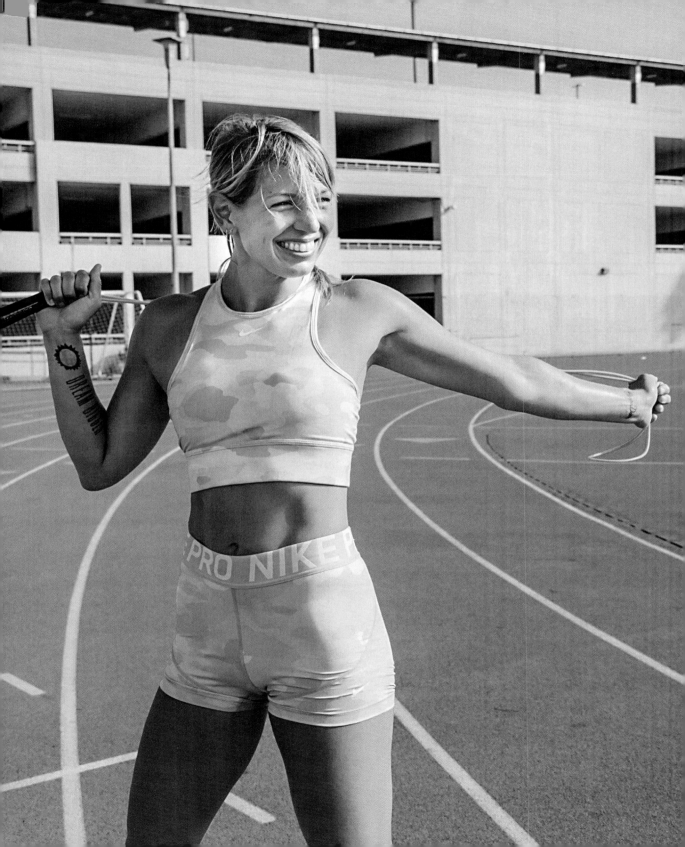

ABOUT THE AUTHOR

KRISTA STRYKER is an NSCA-Certified Personal Trainer and a leading expert on high-intensity interval training (HIIT) and bodyweight fitness. She has helped tens of thousands of people to unlock their full athletic potential through her 12 Minute Athlete blog and fitness app.

Growing up in a super-athletic family, Krista played team sports early on but felt like the athletic gene had skipped her. She never even attempted a push-up until she was in college, when her brother—who called her "Spaghetti Arms"—challenged her to do one. As she struggled through that first push-up, she realized that with hard work and dedication, she too had the potential to become an athlete.

Within a few years, she became certified as a personal trainer and started working long hours in a popular New York City gym. She diligently tried all kinds of fitness programs—running, cardio, weight training, sports-specific training, and cross training—but ended up overtrained, injured, and exhausted, without ever seeing the results she wanted. Then she discovered HIIT training, and everything changed.

Krista developed a system of workouts that could be done in little space, with few pieces of equipment, and in the shortest time possible. Best of all, they actually worked—for her *and* her clients. Before long, Krista was doing feats of exercise she never thought possible, such as pull-ups, handstands, and one hundred burpees in six minutes flat.

From "Spaghetti Arms" to handstand push-ups, Krista is living proof of her philosophy that everybody is an athlete. In addition to her NSCA-CPT, she competes as an amateur boxer and holds a Kettlebell Concepts certification, a Yellow Belt in Krav Maga, and a World Calisthenics Organization certification, and is a Precision Nutrition Certified

Coach. Her work has been featured in the *New York Post* and the *Washington Post*, and on Bodybuilding.com and ESPN.

Krista has lived all over the world, including Amsterdam, New York City, and San Francisco. She currently resides in Venice Beach, California, with her husband, Brian; her dog, Rocket; and her cat, Fishstick. When she isn't doing something fitness-related, you can find her reading a good book, going to music festivals, or traveling the world.

You can find out more about Krista and her work at 12minuteathlete.com. *The 12-Minute Athlete* is her first book.

Get the App!

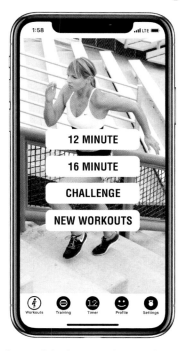

Now that you've learned the basics, take your fitness regimen to the next level with the 12 Minute Athlete HIIT Workouts app.

Available on Google Play and the App Store.

Learn more at
12minuteathlete.com/app